"Thank you for educating me on this topic. Nutrition for the elderly is an important issue, one that we have not paid enough attention to. I will do my best to inform my colleagues in the legislature on this issue."

—**Florida State Senator Nancy Detert**
Committee for Children, Families and Elder Affairs

"As a speech pathologist and amateur cook I find *Essential Purée: The A to Z Guidebook* by Diane Wolff deliciously wonderful. All members of a family can have a nutritional meal that tastes great and can meet diet consistency restrictions. Purée diets no longer need to be bland or boring. This book will be a reference for both my patients and my family."

—**David Fagen, M.A., CCC-SLP, Speech-Language Pathologist**

"As a registered dietitian, I understand the importance of good nutrition and hydration to promote health and wellness. Oftentimes, when a person has impaired swallowing function, it becomes very challenging to maintain necessary nutrient and fluid levels. This book provides many creative tips and tricks to incorporate fresh fruits and vegetables, herbs and sauces into the puréed diet. A cookbook devoted to purée friendly 'comfort food' fills a void in the cookbook world and is well overdue."

—**Kathleen Oliver, RD, LD/N Director of Foodservice, Morrison Healthcare**

"Just like you wouldn't put diesel in your gasoline engine car, you shouldn't put junk in your body either. Healthy nutrition is essential whether you can chew or not. I have been fortunate enough to try Diane's scrumptious meals over the years while I was treating her ailing mother. In one word: marvelous!"

—**Csongor Daniel, author of** *Biotherapy: A Healing for the 21st Century* **and**
The Girl with the Healing Hands

"Getting to know Diane during the 27 years I managed the health food store that she frequents, I've come to respect her commitment to health and vitality using the best of ingredients, most of them organic. These recipes, complete with tips, are not just for those with medical needs but also for those interested in healthy puréed meal on the go – delicious and convenient."

—**Craig Marquis, Richard's Foodporium.**

"Thanks for your work in this often overlooked area."

—Leeza Gibbons
Leeza Gibbons Memory Foundation

"As a neurologist I treat many diseases that affect swallowing. Patients often require a puréed diet and suffer from a decreased appetite and poor nutrition. This book offers great suggestions to make puréed food nutritious and tasty."

—Amy Mellor, MD

"Following dental surgery, my patients are often restricted to a soft diet for a few days up to several weeks. During this time, it is important that they have adequate nutrition to promote successful healing. "Essential Purée" is an excellent resource for patients to maintain their nutritional needs with options that are flavorful and delicious."

—Joseph C. Bender, D.M.D.

"As a Dermatologic Surgeon specializing in skin cancer treatment, I frequently recommend a soft diet for patients after having surgery near the mouth or jaw. Until now, I could never be specific about what type of "soft diet" to prepare. With Diane Wolff's new book, "Essential Purée: The A to Z Guidebook", I now have a wonderful reference for my patients. Not only does this book provide ideas for my recommended diet, it does so in a healthy and delicious way! The book is well-written and easy to follow, and I endorse it not only for my patients, but also for their family members with a taste for nutritional comfort food, prepared in a unique and creative fashion!"

—Jay S. Herbst, M.D.
Dermatologic Surgeon, Director, South Florida Skin Center

"This book is such a great resource for us."

—Donna Gajewski, R.N.
Director of Clinical Services, Nurse On Call Home Health Care

"Mrs. Grossman loved the food. She looked forward to her meals and had a good appetite. She always enjoyed her food and functioned well on the diet. Everything worked."

—Beatrice Marie Castlejean, CNA
Aide to Cathie Grossman for five years

67 GOURMET RECIPES FOR A SOFT DIET

ESSENTIAL
PURÉE

THE A TO Z GUIDEBOOK

DIANE WOLFF

Printed in the United States of America

Revised Edition, June 2016
First Printing, July 2015

ISBN: 978-0-692-44517-4

EssentialPuree.com

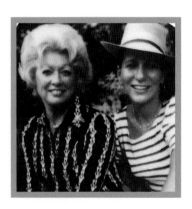

Dedicated to the memory of my mother,
Cathie Grossman

"Good cooking is no mystery. You don't need years of culinary training, or rare and costly foodstuffs or an encyclopedic knowledge of world cuisines. You need only your own senses. You need good ingredients, too."

Alice Waters
Proprietor of Chez Panisse Restaurant
Founding mother of the California food revolution
from *The Art of Simple Food*

CONTENTS

From Here On In, It's All Purée
Creative Solutions for Caregivers and Families

The Essential Purée Guidebook is an emergency response guide for caregivers of patients with swallowing difficulties. I come from a family of great cooks and have traveled all over the world looking for great food and great stories. This is the book I wish I had when my mother developed swallowing difficulties.

From the moment of diagnosis of dysphagia or swallowing difficulties, suddenly the diet is all purée. This may sound simple, but it is not. I was my mother's principal caregiver. When she received the diagnosis of swallowing difficulties, I kicked into high gear.

I researched the available cookbooks, experimented with brands of products that were commercially available. I tried out kitchen tools. I consulted healthcare professionals in all the medical fields and found resources, where to order such things as thickened water and thickened ice cream. This took time, months and years. I gathered all of that experience into one easy-to-use how-to guidebook.

The Guidebook incorporates many tips and tricks. It takes the caregiver step by step through the setup, organization and use of a purée kitchen. It also suggests how to cook on a schedule, how many portions to cook at one time, how to store food safely, how to label the food, and how to purée it for the perfect texture for ease of swallowing of the patient.

Most of what is commercially available off the shelf is boring, tasteless and loaded with harmful ingredients as well as preservatives and chemicals. This guidebook tells how to prepare delicious food simply and easily, cheaper and better than commercially available products. The 67 recipes in the Guidebook are family recipes that have been prepared for years. They are updated versions of classic American comfort foods done in a healthy balanced manner.

The Guidebook contains a product review of kitchen tools and appliances to set up the purée kitchen and get the home cook or the institutional cook up and running. The resource section of the Guidebook tells where to order thickening products, in stores and online.

Setting up a purée kitchen means the cook needs an organizational guide to pantry, fridge and freezer. A cooking schedule is a must. Cooking in batches is a must. A shopping guide is a must. One does not want to be chained to the kitchen. Organization is your best tool to always have a delicious and nutritious meal on hand. This Guidebook removes the guesswork.

This book is for caregivers and family members, but it is also for the institutional cook who may not be getting the desired result with purée prepared for patients. The big secret to the art of purée is: the sauce is the medium of flavor. The rules for purée are different than simply liquefying a meal prepared for the general patient.

This guidebook can also be used by the person in good health who wants a nutritious meal on the go. This could be for reasons of convenience or time, for work or for travel, or for the gym. It is for road warriors and busy moms everywhere, and for the fitness-minded who have no appetite for the fast food life.

Let me tell you how this guidebook came to be. My mother, Cathie Grossman, was in her eighties. She was generally healthy, but she had begun coughing when she ate and was taking a very long time to eat.

Jenine, one of my mother's home health care aides, said that perhaps my mom needed a swallow test. She also worked in a nursing home and she recognized the problem. We took Cathie G to the doctor. He referred her to a speech-language pathologist (SLP) for evaluation.

The test took an hour. My mom was diagnosed with dysphagia. The word means "difficulty in swallowing" (from the Greek roots dys—difficulty and phagia—to eat).

Dysphagia impacts people of all age groups and is present as a consequence of a number of medical conditions, including age, disease, accident, or, in some cases, as the result of war injuries.

It is widespread. The condition affects a million people a year, according to the CDC. The condition is life-threatening.

Feeding is basic to life. The patient has to eat or the patient will die. If the patient coughs and aspirates food, they can get bacterial pneumonia. It is difficult to cure and requires hospitalization. It is, potentially, life-threatening.

The doctor informed us that from that moment forward, my mother would eat puréed food.

BOOM! The change was instantaneous. It happened all of a sudden. If you are reading this book and coping with this situation, you know the situation.

I was confronted by a dilemma. What was I to do? My challenge was to adapt my cooking to purée. I stepped up to the challenge, motivated by love for my mother. I wanted her to have a good old age. I did not want her to lose quality of life.

Being an author, I did what I always do. I went into high-performance mode. I did my homework. I did the research. I was determined to get on top of the situation. I interviewed every professional health care giver in every specialty. I consulted every cookbook available.

I went through a period of trial and error. I looked for meals, puréed products that were available commercially. I got them home and tasted them. I found nothing that was tasty.

It was suggested by an R. N. of our acquaintance that I try puréed baby foods, but baby digestion and nutrient requirements are not the same as for adults. Besides, the baby food was tasteless and had chemicals and preservatives in them. That's why mothers of all ages are making their own baby food to get better quality into the building blocks of their babies' future health.

I had a well-equipped kitchen, but I was cooking constantly to get food for my mom. I had to find a more efficient system and the right tools to give me the right result. This naturally took some time and some experimentation.

I researched every cookbook available but none of them was adequate. Some were exotic, some did not have good instructions. This guidebook contains tips, tricks, and secrets to making great tasting purée.

The health care professionals said the same thing. Nutrition for the elderly was a completely overlooked area. It was a national scandal. There was nothing really good on the market. From the CNAs to the dietitians and speech pathologists to the doctors in many specialties, all of them knew there was a need in the marketplace but none of them knew what to do about it.

I realized that if my mother were to have a healthy diet, I could not buy it in the store. It was up to me. That is how this guidebook came about.

The great physicians of medical traditions, East and West, agree that food is medicine. Increasingly the general public has become aware of the importance of nutrition in maintaining good health, even into advanced age. The idea of nutritional healing is taking hold in our time. You can affect your health through food. Food contains the building blocks of cells and of life.

The recipes in this book are the basics of a classic American tradition, done in an updated and healthy manner. I am broadening out my scope with the new recipes being posted on our website (EssentialPuree.com) to include global cuisine, with contributions from many food cultures. For now, I encourage anyone of any cultural heritage to use the principles of this guidebook to create purée from classic recipes of their own traditions. Just remember, the sauce is the secret to great purée.

Flavor, flavor, flavor is the first principle of this guidebook. Variety is the second principle. A great American cook, the Barefoot Contessa, says that all a really good cook needs to know are 10 great recipes. Then you work on the variation. This is simple for any home cook. Neither the cook nor the patient wants to get stuck in a rut. The way out of the rut is to know your classic flavor profiles and use healthy ingredients. With this approach, you can create endless variety. Know what is possible.

The Essential Purée approach: You can greatly influence one's health and prevent disease simply by eating well. This is called nutritional healing. This approach has created a regular tsunami in the food world.

The rage for nutritional healing is everywhere. Famous chefs are opening new restaurants that focus on healthy eating and organic products. From the Doctor Oz show to prominent fitness trainers such as Jillian Michaels to former supermodels with cable TV shows, such as Carole Alt; to doctors of integrative medicine with shows on PBS, to infomercials dedicated to nutrition extraction machines, it seems that cleaning up the diet is recognized as the way to good health.

The ancient principle of food as medicine is new again. In other words, perfectly healthy people might choose to eat puréed foods for reasons of convenience, health, and fitness.

Example: The seasonal smoothie: Sometimes on a cold morning, one does not want a cold smoothie. A warm smoothie is soothing, even before the gym. The new tools allow you to make a hot smoothie, not quite a soup, but not quite raw. Warms the tummy on a cold morning.

Example: A friend of mine had a plastic surgery procedure, a facelift, and could not eat solid food for a week. I printed out a copy of my cookbook manuscript; she made the puréed food and drank it through a straw. It got her through the post-op recovery period.

Example: The manager of my whole foods store recommended the cookbook to someone who had had gastric bypass surgery as a means of getting control of obesity. He used the cookbook to get him through the post-op period.

Example: An investment banker friend of mine was always taking a plane to some far corner of the world. He was tired of eating airplane food, airport meals, and take-out sandwiches. He wanted to take good food with him in a portable container and eat it as a purée.

He wanted to eat it cold in summer and microwaved in winter as hot food. He wanted it packed in portable containers that would not open in his briefcase. For the road warrior in him, the puréed meal was a salvation.

He liked the no fuss. He liked that a good meal on the go saved him mental energy—he did not have to think about getting food in airports. It was a time-saver. It was high quality and clean eating.

The third principle of this Guidebook is flexibility and adaptation. In this, I follow the great chef Julia Childs, who says that the context determines the menu. I use convenience foods and high-quality store-bought foods and keep them in the pantry for the days when I cannot find the time to shop. When the pantry is well-stocked, there is always a meal on hand.

Once in a while if my mom had a craving for a burger from MacDonald's I found a way to purée it, with special sauce, ketchup, and pickle. Why not? Why be rigid? A little extra special sauce, a little extra ketchup, some water, only half the bun and you have a Big Mac purée. Improvisation is a great thing. Julia Childs famously said that when on the road, eat road food. Don't be a food snob.

As another example of improvisation: Think outside the box. I used a deconstructed forms of my mom's favorite foods. In particular, she liked banana cream pie. I realized that I did not have to make a whole pie if it was going to be puréed. I went for taste. I assembled all the elements and worked on getting beautiful texture. I could create several servings and did not have to throw out uneaten food. One does not want to waste in the kitchen.

This cookbook employs a fourth principle, that of the great Zen Buddhist chefs. There are simple everyday foods which we eat most of the time and then there are feast foods which we eat on special occasions. For the most part, this guidebook focuses on simple food elevated to the level of fabulous. It also includes recipes for holidays.

There is no reason that puréed food cannot be festive and carry the familiar flavors of Thanksgiving and Christmas. My traditional dish for New Year's Day brunch is lobster pot pie. It is casual but elegant and it is a celebration by virtue of being luxurious. The recipe is included in the section on Entrees.

For this guidebook I use the diets recommended by the American Heart Association, the National Dysphagia Diet from the American Dietetic Association and also that of the American Diabetic Association. I also consulted and used the Department of Agriculture's the Choose My Plate guidelines.

The food is low fat, low salt and low sugar. I use lean protein, fresh fruits and vegetables, and whole grains. I use great quality ingredients. I use organic foods when possible and whole foods, meaning foods with as little processing as possible, and without chemical additives and preservatives. This is simply Clean Eating.

The idea of nutritional healing goes back thousands of years, in the medical traditions of East and West. The great chef and founder of the California food revolution, Alice Waters, advocates eating locally, eating seasonally and eating sustainably. This philosophy of food as medicine is in complete agreement with the founder of Western medicine Hippocrates and the ancient wisdom of traditional Chinese medicine.

This book is for all of the people who inhabit the realm of the sick and those who inhabit the realm of the healthy. Essential Purée is for the healthy person who wants a nutritious meal on the go. These people want to escape fast foods and vending machines.

This guidebook speaks to another trend: millions of people are currently making raw foods smoothies made with nutrition extractor blenders. Essential Purée takes the idea a step further. The Essential Purée recipes may be used for the cooked smoothie, a healthy portable meal in liquid form.

I learned how to cook at my mother's side, doing small kitchen tasks to help with family meals. With time, mother and daughter reversed roles. I used to tell my mom that it was a lucky thing that she was such a good mother and taught me how to cook, for everything she taught me how to cook, I was now cooking for her.

I salute the caregivers, for it is very easy to become burned out or isolated. This Guidebook offers the insight that the sharing of food has a way of creating a community and the circle expands. I started out cooking for my mother and I wound up cooking for a widening circle of family, employees, and friends.

"Life is too precious and far too short to eat boring tasteless food" is my personal motto and the motto of this cookbook.

I do this work in my mother's memory. I dedicate this book to my mother, the late great Cathie G, a great lady and a great role model. I think she would have loved the idea that what was created for her could be of benefit to others.

Please consult the patient's primary caregiver as to the suitability of Essential Purée recipes for each individual patient. This is especially true for raw foods.

A note about desserts: Patients who are diabetic should substitute dessert recipes from a diabetic cookbook, but apply the Essential Purée principles of how to get the perfect purée.

Cooking is creative. If you have the right tools, it is never a chore. I do a short product review in Chapter 2 and an updated product review on EssentialPuree.com.

Setting Up the Purée Kitchen
Basic Tools and Techniques

In our day, nutritional healing is being recognized as an important part of health and healing. This brings purée into the contemporary world. The country at large is undergoing a new consciousness of the importance of nutrition in maintaining good health throughout life. Nutrition for the elderly should be a national priority.

Here is the step by step guide to setting up a kitchen for making puréed food, whether for medical reasons or for reasons of healthy eating on the go. There are secrets to getting flavor into purée and this book tells you how.

Rule of Thumb:

The most important labor-saving device is organization. It simplifies the job in a home health care setting.

The rules and tips in this section hold true for the chef in a healthcare institution. As many institutional cooks discovered, puréeing regular food often means loss of flavor. The rules apply to home health care situations as well as healthcare facilities.

Stock the pantry. Keep great ingredients on hand for the too busy to shop day. Get the right ingredients. Shop your neighborhood. Know your sources, the best farmer's market, the best fishmonger, the best supermarket. Know where to get the best ingredients locally and sustainably.

Get the right tools. Use the product review guide to help you get the right tools at the right price, most importantly, that fit into your kitchen space. Set up the tools for ease of access.

Know what to cook and how to cook it.

Shop on a schedule. Cook on a schedule. Set aside the right days when you have time to do the job. Make sure the schedule is easy and convenient. If you have time, cook two dishes on a single cooking day.

Cook in Batches of four to six Servings. This saves time and money. It also simplifies cleanup.

Get the right containers for food storage and the right materials for food labeling food.

Portion and Label the Food: For Immediate Use. One portion served on the day the dish is cooked. One portion goes in the fridge for service that week. Two go in the freezer for use within a month.

Follow simple rules for food safety. See the food safety website. Do not leave food sitting out for more than two hours. Refrigerate.

Keep a White Board. List Entrees and Side Dishes and Sauces on one board. Desserts, Salads, and Fruit Sauces on a second board.

Healthful Cooking Techniques

These are baking, roasting, grilling, steaming, stir fry and pan sautéing.

When the cook has time or has a work day, the slow cooker is convenient. When the cook is in a hurry, the new pressure cookers are a real time savor and preserve nutrients and flavor.

You will not find recipes for deep fry in this cookbook. Too difficult to purée to a smooth texture.

The Right Tools

For the first two years, I cooked for my mother, I used my kitchen as it was set up, a cooktop, an oven, regular pots and pans. The two most basic tools for the purée kitchen are the mini food processor (3.5 cup model) and a good blender. I have several different models of this handy tool. The reason I like it is that it enables the cook to purée one or two servings.

If you are doing very large batches for a healthcare facility, you will probably need a food processor with a large cup capacity.

I like the flat-bottomed blenders with the double row of blades. The Ninja is my favorite.

As I began cooking in batches I added a rice cooker, a three-tiered steamer, a grill and griddle, a multi-cooker, a Ninja four-in-one cooker, an electric wok and an induction burner with a flat-bottomed wok. My most recent acquisitions are an electric pressure cooker and a Ming Tsai turbo-convection cooker. Both render a moist texture while retaining flavor.

The high speed commercial blenders such as the Vitamix, the NutriBullet Rx and the NutriNinja are so powerful that they liquefy many proteins, fruits and vegetables with ease. Some have heat functions for making soups in a blender on a seven-minute cycle.

The nutrition extractors such as the NutriBullet are an excellent tool in the purée kitchen. By breaking down fruits and vegetables, they release the all-important phytochemicals.

I adopted these tools for three reasons: convenience, labor-saving, time-saving and money-saving, in addition to easy cleanup. All were made of good materials.

The rice cooker, slow cooker, electric pressure cooker, four-in-one cooker and electric wok are good for batch cooking. They will make four to six servings with no problem.

The three-tiered steamer will steam an entire head of broccoli or cauliflower. Texture is important for purée. This appliance steams evenly, the best result I have ever had in steaming. It is useful for a quickie meal. It is possible to place a steam packet of a piece of fish or chicken, seasonings, cooked rice and vegetable, and steam the whole packet for purée. Fast and easy.

These kitchen appliances are versatile. They may be used indoors or outdoors and for travel.

The Five Tools For Making Perfect Purée

The High Speed Commercial Blender
The Vitamix, the Nutribullet Rx or the NutriNinja are three of the most popular varieties. These have very powerful motors and very sharp, specially engineered blades. They have the capacity of breaking down cell walls of ingredients to achieve a completely smooth consistency. This includes whole grains such as rice and quinoa.

The Pressure Cooker
These have the ability to reduce protein to a smooth moist texture in a shorter amount of cooking time. (When I refer to a pressure cooker, I mean one of the new electric pressure cookers that are computerized and completely safe. I am not referring to the old-fashioned stovetop pressure cookers that are so scary.)

The Potato Ricer
Once a vegetable is pressure cooked, or cooked by any other method that renders it tender, such as steaming, the potato or the hard squash or the soft beet, can be put through the potato ricer. This creates small grain-like textures that can then be mashed with milk or broth or any other cooking liquid for a smooth purée. The potato ricer is a press that holds a cup of potatoes that have been cooked to tender. The potato goes in the holder, the handle is pressed down, the potato comes out like grains of soft-cooked rice. This produces velvet-y mashed potatoes when combined with butter and milk or cream.

The Food Mill

This is the staple gadget of the French housewife. It is used for eliminating any roughness of texture from any vegetable ingredient or any soup or sauce. You put a small amount of food in the well of the cone shape and you twirl the handle. A blade circulates, forcing the food through a sieve, leaving behind large particles that will not go through the sieve. The milled food has a very smooth texture with no lumps. This produces the most glorious gravies and sauces.

The Mesh Sieve and Silicone Spatula

Put any food item that has been puréed in a food processor or a blender through the mesh sieve with the metal spatula and any and all particles not suitable will be left behind. The sieve can also be lined with cheesecloth. This is especially good for removing the seeds from fruits such as strawberries, raspberries and kiwi.

Cook in Batches of Four to Six Servings

Making multiple servings lightens the cooking schedule.

One always has a meal on hand ready to serve. This is excellent if one is detained or away for a period of time. Food service continues on schedule without the cook's presence on site.

The recipes are for four to six servings. This keeps the refrigerator and freezer stocked.

One serving is puréed for same day service. One serving goes in the fridge, with a label, in a glass storage container with a lid, labeled for service during the week.

The other two servings are labeled and frozen for use within a month.

Follow Basic Rules for Food Safety

Food in the fridge has an expiration date of four days to maximum one week. In the case of seafood, three days is the maximum.

Food in the freezer has a 30-day expiration date. If the date goes by, pitch the food. No exceptions. No questions. This was the rule in the house.

Keep Track of What You Have On Hand

Keep the White Board posted on the freezer current. That way, you know what you have on hand, you know what you need to prepare.

In the interest of preserving the maximum amount of flavor, I froze the dish in its cooked state and puréed the dish only at the time of service. It is fine to purée and store in fridge and freezer, if this suits your household routine.

Making the Purée

There are a number of kitchen appliances for making the purée. I recommend the best for getting good texture.

When I first set up the purée kitchen, I used a blender that contained a well with the blades in the bottom and a screw off removable bottom. I soon realized that this machine was difficult to clean. Food got stuck beneath the blades. Even though the bottom came out, food got stuck. One set of blades did not give the desired consistency of a smooth purée.

A flat-bottomed blender with several layers of blades did a better job, I soon discovered. This was the Ninja. I rate many of the blenders on the market in the product review section, chapter two and in an ongoing manner, on the website. The blender is important. You will use it multiple times per day. Make sure you have a good one.

I used the Nutribullet for maximum extraction of phytochemicals so necessary to good health, including the antioxidants and anti-inflammatory compounds found in fresh fruit and vegetables.

The Big Secret

The big secret to Essential Purée is the sauce. The cook needs good sauces, homemade and prepared. Why, you may ask?

Protein does not purée smoothly without a medium to support the smaller particles.

Essential Purée uses gravy, sauce, soup, and vegetable purée (mashed potato, mashed sweet potato or mashed turnip, butternut squash, the very delicious kabocha or any other winter squash) as great mediums for purée. They add color, nutrients and texture.

My mother liked sweets, so I learned to use ice cream to purée desserts like pies and cakes. I also use fruit sauces for puréeing pancakes and pies.

My mother liked fresh fruit and I include instructions on how to purée melons and other favorites of hers. A note on seeds: Any food containing seeds or particles has to be strained for the patient who has difficulty in swallowing. This includes kiwi and strawberries.

The Best Texture: Make Sure the Purée is Smooth

I took to using white pepper because the particles of black pepper caused my mother to cough. I did not use mozzarella cheese in cooking lasagna, for I did not want the strings of cheese to cause swallowing problems.

Patients must follow the guidelines of the speech pathologist in observing the individual swallowing routine. Please consult your healthcare professional for instructions.

The three best instant thickeners for food and beverages are ThickenUp Clear, Thick & Easy Clear and Simply Thick. For a variety of drinks, the SloDrinks products are excellent. See the Resources Section at the back of this book for more information.

One very important point: All liquids must be thickened without exception. I did not realize at first that my mother's oral dental rinse and her liquid medications such as cough medicine had to be thickened. This is easy to overlook and may cause complications.

Guidebook Recipes for the Whole Family

This volume may be used in a home healthcare setting to feed the person with swallowing difficulties as well as the rest of the family. My banker wanted to use the recipes in the book to eat in a more healthy manner, so he could be in better shape for his kids.

The CNAs, home health care aides who came from the agency to help take care of my mom, would ask me if they could taste the food when the smells started wafting through the house. Of course I fed them. I wanted them to taste the food so that they would know what they were feeding my mother.

I know from practical experience that the clean eating, nutritional healing and healthful cooking influence rubbed off on all those around me. One of the assistants started cooking Guidebook recipes and stopped going to fast-food joints. She dropped two dress sizes over a period of months. She feels terrific.

Michelle, one of our aides from Jamaica, asked for my recipe for sautéed spinach with shallots and garlic recipe so she could make it at home. Her son liked the dish.

Another of our aides had a daughter who was a high school track star. The young woman needed a snack after running because she had to get some carbs into her. The mother tasted the minestrone and made it at home. The daughter liked the minestrone so much that she learned to make it on her own and started taking soup with her to track meets. She also devoured bowls of it when she came home from her track practice.

The daughter went on to win a state championship and was awarded an athletic scholarship to attend college. We made a joke of it and gave some small amount of credit to my minestrone. Even a star athlete must eat for performance. Essential Purée provided the fuel for a young career.

What to Cook?
Classic American Comfort Foods

I wrote this guidebook because of a comment made to me by Suzette, one of the aides who cared for my mother. A former New Yorker of Jamaican descent, she had worked in nursing homes.

She told me that a lot of the elderly who live in nursing homes don't want to eat the food. They lose their appetites, because most puréed foods served in institutions have no taste. Aging for them meant that they lost one of life's greatest pleasures, eating good food. I thought this was so sad.

One has to get nutrition into the patient who is on the purée diet. If the patient does not eat and drops weight, he or she will weaken and will not have the reserve strength to fight off infection. The patient, without proper nutrition, will wither on the vine.

The food I created for my mother was full of flavor. Anyone could do it. If it could help my mother, it could help others.

Food for the Soul

My approach was to use classic American comfort foods with adventurous dishes thrown in for holiday meals and special occasions such as birthdays. Call it American Bistro, the essence of American casual and family dining updated, modernized, and healthy.

I chose mainstream American comfort foods because they represent the every day. They are beloved. They are recognizable. I urge the reader of this book to creatively adapt any comfort foods that come from an ethnic background belonging to the patient in question.

Familiar flavor profiles stimulate the appetite and keep the patient connected to life. The taste of the familiar sets off the pleasure response in the brain.

Food for the Eye

The problem with puréed food is that it all looks the same. To see it is to think of a bowl of oatmeal. This could be boring in the extreme. I offer a solution as to how to get around this problem for the purée patient.

I involved my mother in the process of creating the food. When I returned from the veggie stand, I brought in the eggplant, the papaya, the fresh fruits, the onions, and sweet potatoes and let her see the ingredients that would become her food.

While I was cooking, the smells wafted through the house. This was a stimulant to the appetite. It was a harbinger of good food to come.

When I finished a dish, I brought it into her bedroom and showed it to her. I let her smell it. She ate with her eyes and with her sense of smell before she tasted the purée. She was involved in the process of the preparation and plating of the food, in where the food came from and how it was made.

While this process of involvement is not always possible in an institutional setting, images of the ingredients could be photographed and displayed on a smart TV. In a nursing home, staff could Google and find stock images of the dish and display it on a flat panel screen. The ingredients could even be arranged in a bowl in a public area and put on display. The puréed dish would be the final act in the production.

Food for the Palate

After the cook chooses ingredients for the sake of nutrition, flavor is the most important element in the meal. I cannot stress enough the importance of good sauces and gravies. That is the big secret to great purée. The sauce imparts the velvet mouth feel. This is the essence of the technique: great ingredients, healthy cooking methods, sauce as the medium of flavor.

The sauce allows the proteins to be blended the perfect consistency for swallowing. Fresh ingredients and fresh herbs make a huge difference in flavor. My use of vegetables mashed, such as white potato, sweet potato, butternut squash, or even turnips, as a medium for blending the purée is critical to getting the right texture for the proteins. My use of whole grains gives the all-important fiber to the patient.

Getting the texture right is simple, so simple that it is easily overlooked. Many institutional cooks simply purée the dish served to the rest of the patients. This does not work because of a simple fact of food science. If I season a piece of fish, it tastes good. If I purée the fish, I increase the surface area by a factor of thousands. One could not add enough spice to flavor the protein alone. It would choke the patient. The sauce must carry the flavor.

Often the simplest things are the most difficult. You can't cheat. You either get it or you don't. Perfect your sauces and your purées will be outstanding. Class dismissed.

The Freshest Ingredients
Shop As If Your Life Depended On It, Because It Does

Great-tasting food starts with great ingredients. Making food at home with great ingredients and great cooking methods is cheaper and better. Save money while eating well.

Something to think about: One of the great chefs of the Zen Buddhist cooking tradition (called *kaiseki ryori*) is famously quoted as saying, "Your food becomes your eyes."

So when he suggests rinsing your rice three times until the water comes clear, I do it. In keeping with this idea, I present the fifth guiding principle of Essential Purée: Shop as if your life depends on it, because it does.

In other words, know thy ingredients and thy spices. My advice: Get a black belt in shopping. Be a discerning food consumer.

You would be surprised how willing purveyors are to assist a customer who cares. If you have a question, find someone in the store to ask. Get the manager of the produce department or the head of the seafood department. Ask for their knowledge. They will be delighted to educate and inform you.

This leads me to the sixth guiding principle of Essential Purée, with a nod to Alice Waters: Eat the Neighborhood. Eat locally. Eat in season. Don't go for the exotic, just because it is possible in this age of foods jetted in from every corner of the globe.

I take you on a journey of my neighborhood, with the hope that it inspires you to take a journey through your neighborhood. My home of Florida is an agricultural state with a ten-month growing season. I'm lucky.

The farm stand out on State Road 776 is called Clemon's and it has terrific fruits and vegetables.

Not all the produce is organic, but some of it is. Most of it is locally grown, or the proprietors can tell you where they bought a particular shipment of fabulous-tasting tomatoes or a delivery of papaya, avocado, and starfruit. I shop at this stand for precisely that inside information. I want to know where my fruits and vegetables came from.

I know that the fruits and vegetables on sale have not been held hostage in a refrigerated storage facility, as with the produce at big supermarkets.

The wonders of the botanical world have time to ripen before they come to the store. With light and air and correct temperatures, they mature. They have better flavor.

The clerks admonish you when you go to the tomato carousel with its six or eight varieties of tomatoes. They tell the other customers, not me: Don't squeeze the tomatoes. Go gently.

Where I live on Florida's Gulf Coast, I am close to the Everglades, which produces the most delicious tomatoes in the world. It is the soil, unique to that environment, unique in the world. I will admit that I am prejudiced.

This vegetable stand caters to a wide variety of customers, so I can buy very good fresh shiitake mushrooms, for example, and a wide variety of vegetables used in the Asian kitchen such as baby bok choy and fresh winter melon. I can also buy items from the Latin kitchen, such as various types of peppers.

The historic town of Punta Gorda has a Farmer's Market every weekend during tourist season where one can buy local produce and honey. It's a neighborly place and I go early because Mr. Han, the Chinese-American greengrocer, has the best produce at the Farmer's Market. I want to get first pick. He has a devoted following of customers who have the same idea that I do, and we all know each other because we see each other every weekend.

The Gulf of Mexico is the native abode of the stone crab, for my money the best crab in the world. But again, I have to admit to being prejudiced. When I lived in California, my favorite was the Dungeness crab.

I have found that the organic fruits and vegetables that I buy in the whole foods store often last longer than the fruits and vegetables bought in the supermarket. They are a bit more costly, but I find that because of the longer shelf life, I use more of them and this makes up for the premium in price. Also, the flavor is better. Some items are best when organic, such as apples, pears, grapes, and berries. Others may be bought non-organic, if expense is an issue.

My supermarket has an organic vegetable section. I get better prices shopping in the whole foods store than in the supermarket.

These are the building blocks of the recipes. Begin with good ingredients, use simple cooking techniques, create delicious food.

I buy a beautiful piece of halibut or cod, and all it needs to be superb is a squeeze of lemon juice, a sprinkle of very good olive oil, a little salt and white pepper, the proper grilling. A mouthful of ocean. Perfection!

I keep an eagle eye on quality and an eagle eye on price, and I juggle the two to put the best possible food on the table.

Another rule in the kitchen: Do not waste food. Take a hint from the great chefs: Use Everything. The secrets of nature are in bones and stems, berries and trimmings, shells and stalks. In the kitchen, one gets close to the secrets of life on planet earth.

If I trim the stems off vegetables to get a soft purée, I use the trimmings to make stock, freezing it for later use in small batches. I peel and steam the stems of broccoli, and add them to vegetable soup. Great flavor and great nutrition.

I freeze chicken carcasses and the carcasses of the little Rock Cornish game hens and also use them to make stock. This is a task greatly facilitated by the use of a pressure cooker.

I freeze the stems of kale and chard to make vegetable stock. I freeze the shells of shrimp and lobster for seafood stock, and use them in the appropriate dishes. These are the bearers of flavor and are used it in making the sauce for my seafood pot pie or my fish chowder.

I see the kitchen as a place of transformation. I see the cook as an alchemist dealing with the very chemistry of life itself down to the level of the cells of these precious human bodies.

One must be fierce in the kitchen. Life is precious. Food is precious. Create and invent. Waste nothing.

The object is to create an atmosphere of health and healing. Atmosphere is everything. Healing begins in the mind.

According to one of the great teachers of Traditional Chinese Medicine, an expert in food as medicine, context is an important part of the meal. First is nutrition, second is preparation and service and third is context.

The classics of Chinese literature are full of stories about Chinese emperors and how they value their cooks. Stories abound where the cook is the bearer of mystical wisdom. One such story contends that a certain cook for a certain emperor never had to sharpen his knife because he never encountered bone. When he cut, he knew where the spaces were. His knife never dulled from encountering opposition. He cut through emptiness. Philosophy in the kitchen: One could see this as a wise approach to life in general.

Fresh Ingredients Always on Hand

These are my classic ingredients for the creation of flavor. These are my staples. Please feel free to expand the list to include ingredients that are important to you and your family.

Bananas	Garlic	Avocados
Lemons and limes	Ginger	Celery
Carrots	Onions	Carrots
Yukon Gold Potatoes	Scallions	Spinach
or Red Jacket Potatoes	Mushrooms	Kale
Sweet Potatoes	Tomatoes	

In the fridge:

Milk	Eggs	Applesauce
Parmesan Cheese	Unsalted Butter	

Starting an Herb Garden

My advice is, for the ultimate in fresh ingredients: grow it yourself.

I make my own pesto and always have six basil plants going so that I may harvest the two cups necessary to make a good batch. I also grow Italian flat leaf parsley, chives, rosemary, and sage. I grow oregano, but it takes over, so I keep it in a peat container. I grow mint and dill. I have terrible luck with thyme, but I keep trying.

Fresh herbs add fantastic flavor to cooking. They are easy and rewarding to grow. You can grow them in a kitchen window, in containers, or in the ground. They require water and filtered, not direct, sunlight. A little plant food such as Miracle-Gro® once a month is important.

It is really satisfying to go outside and pick a handful of basil for a pasta sauce, or pick some fresh parsley to chop finely and add to a soup or sprinkle over a piece of fish.

This is the way it goes. First you start cooking and then you start gardening.

The System
Organizing the Pantry and Freezer

A guiding principle of the purée kitchen is to always have a meal on hand. The way to do this is to keep a well-stocked pantry. Convenience foods of the clean eating variety ease the pressures of a busy work life. It is best not to be a food snob. I like making things from scratch, but sometimes I am just too pressed for time.

The pantry is also important for emergency situations: In the land of hurricanes, the Board of Health gives advice for households whose members have medical needs. Keep two weeks' worth of food, water and meds on hand, in case the lights go out in a storm.

THE PANTRY
Tomato Products
Tomato products are a must: Many of my recipes call for tomato products such as tomato paste, tomato purée, tomato sauce, or diced tomatoes. I use the lower sodium variety. One does not want the patient to become dehydrated. This is life-threatening in the elderly.

My supermarket carries a house brand of organic tomato products. They are delicious. I use them whenever possible. They also have a brand of fire-roasted tomato paste and diced tomatoes. These add a lot of flavor to a dish. I use these products when I make a big pot of homemade sauce on Sunday. I then freeze my sauce in quart containers, usually glass, filled three-quarters full to allow for expansion. One does not want the sauce to explode in the freezer

I keep jars of my favorite store-bought pasta sauce, as well as a couple of jars of good, high-quality Alfredo sauce. (The latter I use as a base for my lemon sauce for my salmon in puff pastry).

When using store-bought tomato sauce for pasta dishes, I use a brand that lists a variety of tomatoes as the first ingredient, either plum or Roma. This sauce has better flavor than commercial sauces that list tomato purée as the first ingredient.

I buy pickled beets as my mother loves pickled beet salad with ranch dressing. I add thin slivers of red onion before purée. I keep a good quality sauerkraut in the fridge, for the occasional purée of vegetarian baked beans, all beef hot dogs with mustard and a little kraut on the side.

Pasta

I keep a variety of pastas, thin spaghetti, linguine, penne, and elbow macaroni for mac and cheese. I prefer whole grain pasta. A new passion is black bean pasta and azuki bean pasta. Both are flavorful additions to pasta dishes and are gluten free.

Legumes

I keep dried peas and French lentils for making my mother's favorite cream of pea soup. I keep garbanzos or chick peas for making hummus when I have the time to cook them in the pressure cooker. I keep the bag containing the ingredients for nine bean soup from the health food store. This I buy in bulk. I know the food does not sit in bags on the shelf for long periods of time.

Whole Grains

I keep long grain brown basmati rice. This is my go-to rice because of the flavor and because it cooks up tender. It does not have a tough husk, as short grain brown rice does. The short grain brown rice was too difficult for my mom to digest.

I use kasha or buckwheat groats for variety in carbohydrates.

For fish cakes, I use Yukon gold potatoes cooked and put through a potato ricer. Puréed sweet potato is a staple item because my mother loves them, so every two weeks, I soft bake four or five of them and make them according to the recipe..

I buy quinoa, the high-protein whole grain from South America. This I use as a side dish or I use it in place of rice to make a pilaf or even stuff peppers or cabbage.

From the whole foods store, I use steel cut oats for oatmeal, the five-minute variety as opposed to the 30-minute variety.

I buy buckwheat pancake mix and keep it in the refrigerator. I use fine corn meal for dredging and for making grits. The texture is better for the purée.

For a quickie soup, I use Thai Kitchen Instant Rice Noodle Soups. I use Garlic and Vegetable and Spring Onion flavors, but leave out the heat packet. I add a couple of shrimp and scallops for the protein, and I use a handful of California mix frozen vegetables for a night when I need an In a Hurry Meal. This purées beautifully.

Thickeners

I keep cornstarch, arrowroot, and Wondraflour for thickening sauces and gravies. I use prepared bread crumbs (organic whole wheat from the natural foods store with Italian seasoning), matzo meal, and panko (Japanese-style bread crumbs) for light breading. These all purée well without granules that irritate the throat and make swallowing difficult.

Food thickeners and the sources for ordering them are in the Resources section at the back of the book and also in the updated Resources section on the website, EssentialPuree.com

Spices

I keep a variety of spices: cumin, oregano, thyme, tarragon, sage, turmeric, curry powder, chili powder, whole peppercorns, Kosher salt, Himalayan salt, and sea salt. Old Bay seasoning is a must for fish and shellfish.

The spice cabinet always has Worcestershire sauce and lower-sodium soy sauce, two flavor powerhouses.

I use several varieties of mustard: yellow mustard, Dijon mustard, Chinese mustard.

I use organic ketchup.

I like the Stubbs' barbecue sauce because it is low in sugar. There are four varieties and all of them are good.

I use a good low-fat mayonnaise or Lemonaise.

For a bit of heat, not too much, I use a touch of Tabasco in my chili.

For desserts, I also keep good quality vanilla extract, cinnamon, cloves, nutmeg, allspice. The classics.

Oils and Vinegars

I buy good quality olive oil in glass bottles and extra virgin olive oil for salads and sauces. I also use cold-pressed oils, the Hain brand, polyunsaturated safflower, and sunflower. I like the high smoke point of grapeseed oil. I use walnut and sesame oils. Corn oil is good but has a distinctive flavor, excellent in corn muffins and corn bread. Veronica, one of my mother's aides who is from Jamaica, introduced me to cooking with coconut oil. I love it.

I use very good quality vinegars as well, including rice vinegar because it is light and has a clean taste without the after-acid burn. I use red wine vinegar and sherry vinegar in moderation.

Sweeteners

Note: I avoid refined white sugar and artificial sweeteners. I use the following.

- Local honey
- Real maple syrup
- Barley malt syrup
- Agave Syrup
- Stevia

THE FREEZER

Fruits: I keep frozen blueberries and strawberries, raspberries, pineapple, black cherry and mango, all for fresh fruit purée. I use a nutrition extractor to liquefy the fruits, including apples and pears. I put all fruit purées through a mesh sieve with a silicone spatula to remove seeds and fibers. When seeds are present or fibers, I line the mesh sieve with a layer of cheesecloth and then use the silicone spatula.

Note: Frozen vegetables and fruits are picked at the height of ripeness and flash frozen and make an excellent choice when fresh is not available. Sometimes the busy cook just cannot make it to the market.

Proteins: I keep frozen cooked shrimp (tail on, but tail removed before purée), frozen scallops, and frozen wild salmon fillets.

More Go-To Items For The Freezer
- Ground Turkey (no antibiotics)
- Chicken Breasts (no antibiotics)
- Chicken Italian Sausage (mild) (no antibiotics)
- Loin of Pork
- Peas

- Chopped Spinach
- Corn
- Southland Puréed Butternut Squash
- Southland Puréed Turnips

Note: You do not have to keep all of these on hand, but pick and choose those you find will fit into your own concept of Essential Purée.

Food Storage

I prefer glass containers with lids, available in sets in Wal-Mart or Target. The glass is more expensive, particularly if you use the type that can go from freezer to microwave, but glass is better for the environment, as plastic does not last long before staining with the sauces. In the alternative, use BPA-free plastic containers in a variety of sizes for entrees, vegetables, fruits, and desserts.

I use Post-It labels, the ruled 4 x 6 size, and I write down the name of the dish, the contents of the dish, the fact that it is one serving, and that the dish needs to be puréed.

I store in single servings, so that there are no bits and pieces of leftovers cluttering up the fridge.

I make a label with the date of preparation of the food, and a "use by" date which is usually 30 days from the date of freezing.

With seafood, I use a two-week date.

When I freeze baked goods, I wrap the baked goods in plastic wrap and then aluminum foil and put it in the plastic or glass container. The pot pie stays very fresh.

I also do this with cupcakes and birthday cake. The bakery lady, Donna, at my Publix supermarket gave me that tip.

Food Safety

I use guidelines for food safety gleaned from the master chefs on the Food Network and also on the Department of Agriculture website.

Food may remain in the refrigerator for four up to seven days. I use three in the case of seafood.

Food may remain in the freezer for up to 30 days. When the dates expire, the food is thrown away.

No questions asked. Out it goes.

Further guidelines may be found on the website for the Food Institute, along with an online tutorial.

THE SYSTEM

How to Keep Track of Meals on Hand and Make a Shopping & Cooking Schedule

To keep track of meals, I used two small white boards and put them on the freezer door. These were the kind that attached with magnets and had a pen holder for the marker. I kept erasers close by.

I updated the boards every time I cooked and stored and every time I used food. The boards told me and any other caregiver what was on hand.

I listed entrees on one board along with soups and veggie side dishes. On the other, I listed salads, desserts, savory and fruit sauces.

I listed the quantity of units in the freezer and kept it up to date with additions and subtractions. That way, I always knew what I had on hand. Other caregivers always knew what was on hand. The patient could select from the items available. Everyone's job was easier.

From the white board, I made a cooking schedule. If I ran out of pea soup, my mother's favorite, I made a batch.

I made up shopping schedules from the white boards. I knew what I needed in terms of fresh ingredients. I used meals that were already cooked before I cooked more. Neither food nor money were wasted with this system.

The system outlined in this guidebook saves labor in the long run. One does not cook too much and one does not cook too little. One does not buy food that one cannot use. One does not waste time and gas running to the market. It is a means of staying on top of the purée kitchen.

Another bonus: You will probably have to use the purée appliance a number of different times a day. The system makes everything more efficient and minimizes cleanup

Melons in the Freezer

My mother loved melon, but she could not eat a half cantaloupe or a quarter of a watermelon or a whole honeydew before the fruit went bad.

I wanted to give my mom plenty of fresh fruit, so I puréed four servings, a serving being a half cup of purée. I used enough fresh fruit to create the four serving batch. The fruit was thickened with instant thickener to her level of the NDD diet. See Instant Thickeners information in the Resources Section.

I divided the batch up. Two servings for the refrigerator and two servings for the freezer. All were in individual containers, labeled and dated, four days in the fridge, two weeks in the freezer.

I mention this as an important part of the system because I emphasize the importance of fresh fruit and vegetables in the Essential Purée Guidebook. Fruit is expensive and one does not want to waste it by allowing it to go bad on the counter or in the fridge.

Batch cooking is a hallmark of the Essential Purée system. Making four to six servings is the secret to success. The batch maximizes the use of the cook's time and energy. One is not chained to the kitchen.

Freezing is essential as it saves money. Nothing goes to waste. Freezing is especially important dealing with large fruit such as papaya, a favorite of my mother's.

I also purée: watermelon, a variety of other melons, pineapple, papaya, mango, and kiwi. (Strain the seeds out of kiwi after puréeing. They are difficult to swallow.)

In season, I purée all types of berries. They are less expensive. I purée grapes and cherries. I pit fresh cherries, of course.

I purée stone fruits such as apricots and peaches, after removing the pit. Apple purées nicely. I purée pear, sometimes after poaching it, but serve it immediately if I want a warm dessert.

I use pomegranate juice for flavor and do not pulverize pomegranate seeds in the nutrition extractor. The seeds have a bitter taste when puréed. They are not pleasant.

Banana is the king of puréed fruits and freezes beautifully. Purée it with a little dried coconut, unsweetened, and you have the basis of a great dessert. A little vanilla ice cream and a little Nocciolatta hazelnut chocolate sauce, with a little fresh cherry fruit sauce and you have a banana sundae in a dish. Straight to purée, without creating the sundae first, a deconstructed dessert. Nocciolatta does not have trans-fats in it.

Thickening Hint for Frozen Fruit

Frozen fruit has to be thickened. That said, it is best to freeze puréed fruit in an unthickened state and thicken before serving. That way, one does not have to freeze the thickening agent.

My favorite product: I used Simply Thick in packets in the nectar consistency or honey consistency, depending on my mother's need at the time. The new thickeners such as Thick It Clear and Thicken Up Clear will freeze when used according to package directions. See Resources for information to order.

A Note Concerning Meatless Proteins

I include meatless variations in some of my recipes.

In my Veggie Chili recipe, I use tempeh, which is a vegetarian protein source from Indonesia made of organic soybeans with millet, brown rice, and barley. This is available in whole foods stores and is manufactured by the LightLife Company, which has been making it for 40 years.

The tempeh comes packaged as a rectangle and can be sliced and diced the way that one would use any protein. The prep is to pan sauté it in a little oil with a dash of soy sauce. For the chili recipe it is browned, as one would brown ground meat, and then added to the recipe.

The LightLife Company also makes an extensive line of meat substitutes that are tasty as well as nutritious and any of these can be substituted for the recipes in this cookbook that call for meat.

I sometimes add non-GMO firm tofu to a soup for extra protein and also for thickening. This is a soy product and should not be used by anyone with a food allergy.

Tofu has been a staple of Chinese and Japanese vegetarian cooking for centuries. It makes an excellent substitute for buttermilk, mayo, and sour cream when making homemade ranch dressing.

Here is the no-recipe recipe for those who like to cook by feel: Use a half cup of oil and a quarter cup of vinegar as your base, add some capers and salt and white pepper and purée in a half cake of tofu. All of this is done to taste. Taste as you go.

Add more tofu, a small amount at a time, to adjust for degree of creaminess desired. Add some chives if you want it to turn green. Tofu ranch dressing keeps in the fridge for two weeks.

Tofu is available in local supermarkets and natural food stores. It has no flavor and takes on the flavor of the dish. Once opened, refrigerate and use within a few days. Water should be changed daily. Think of it as Japanese mozzarella but without the stretchiness.

The Biggest Secret to the Art of Purée
The Sauce

Flavor, flavor, flavor. How to get it? How to keep it?

Here is the biggest secret to the art of purée: The sauce is everything, the medium for carrying flavor. It permeates and surrounds. Think of the ingredients as swimming in the pool of sauce.

If you take away nothing else from this book, you will have the secret of great purée. Getting the flavor is a matter of common sense. There is simple food science behind my approach. When you purée food, you increase the volume of surface area. That is why the food becomes tasteless. You cannot add enough spice to make up for this situation. You will ruin the food. It would not be good for the patient. It would not do the trick.

This is why institutional food has no taste and what prepared puréed food, commercially available, is lacking.

The secret is the sauce. This is not rocket science. The object is to create a smooth purée that tastes great and is easy to swallow.

The way to solve this problem is with a light sauce that improves the texture of the purée and carries the flavor. I am not speaking of old-fashioned sauces made with a roux of flour and butter for these do not purée as well.

Make a great sauce or gravy or soup as a base for your purée and you have a great dish. The idea is to flavor the liquid and let the liquid flavor the food. The liquid wraps around the molecules of food and suddenly the dish is singing with flavor. I cannot emphasize this enough:

The sauce may be tomato sauce, brown gravy, Alfredo sauce, barbecue sauce, or curry. My particular favorite of the moment is any sauce made from a soup that is primarily a vegetable base. The soups can be bought off the shelf if you don't have time for scratch: mushroom, onion, celery, red pepper, butternut squash, even seafood chowder, clean varieties please.

The sauce may be as simple as a broth: chicken broth, vegetable broth, beef broth. Homemade or store-bought. The purée liquid can be water or milk. I don't use heavy cream, but if that suits your palette, cream will purée. Coconut milk, soy milk, almond milk, cashew milk will also do. I use coconut milk of the light variety in my curries—curry sauce, of the mild variety, is a beautiful medium for purée. Watch the saturated fat content when using coconut milk.

The sauce could be a dashi from the Japanese kitchen, such as kombudashi made with dried kombu or kelp. This is very light and works well with seafood.

Flavor and texture are the two most important elements for foolproof purée. The second great task of the sauce is to create a pleasing texture. Without the right amount of liquid, protein becomes grainy. Use the sauce for flavor and then, if necessary, use a mashed vegetable for creaminess of texture and ease of swallowing. Taste as you go. Experiment.

How much sauce is enough? You should have enough liquid in any dish to give the correct consistency for ease of swallowing. I start with a half cup. I adjust from there. If I run short, I follow the advice of the great French chef Jacques Pepin and I use water in small amounts.

As to texture and thickness, this is where experience counts. Taste and test. You will get the hang of it. Observe the patient. The patient's ability to swallow with ease is the absolute guideline. Too thick and it is an effort for the patient to swallow. Too thin and the patient may aspirate the food. The speech pathologist determines the level of the National Dysphagia Diet (NDD). See Resources Section for definitions.

Put yourself in the patient's position. Think of how terrible it must be to have difficulty in getting food down. It must be an exercise in frustration. Have compassion and adjust the thickness of the purée. You will see the patient respond as the swallow becomes easy.

A word of advice: Some foods are prohibited on the National Dysphagia Diet (NDD). Check with your healthcare provider. I use white pepper instead of black pepper because black pepper grains are larger and present a hazard to swallowing. I do not use mozzarella cheese in lasagna because of the stretchy quality of the cheese. Ricotta with parmesan and mascarpone give you creamy protein without the hazard of the stretch.

I use a practical approach to stocking sauces: Although I make many sauces from scratch, I keep some store-bought sauces in the pantry. These are of the highest quality and have the least preservatives. They include my favorite store-bought tomato sauce for pasta, and Alfredo sauce, which I use as a base for the lemon sauce for my salmon cakes. Make sure your store-bought pasta sauce has tomatoes as the first ingredient.

I have on hand at all times soups in paper containers from the health food store: I use organic cream of tomato, cream of celery, cream of mushroom, cream of red pepper and butternut squash soups. These become bases for sauces. They also become bases for soups, by adding protein, carbs and veggies. These days, good brands of these soups also available in the natural foods section of supermarkets.

As I said in the pantry chapter, even great chefs use convenience foods. The purée kitchen is not the place to practice food snobbery nor to be lax and go junk food. Practicality rules supreme. The object is to have great-tasting food available, especially when you have to delegate a meal service.

Be a creative cook. When you make a pot roast, freeze the extra gravy. When freezing liquids, bear in mind that one only fills a freezer container of liquid three-quarters full to allow the liquid to expand when freezing. The extra gravy may be used to purée meat loaf, roast beef, noodles with beef, or any other dish where pot roast gravy would be a match. When storing in containers in freezer, sauce is labeled with a "use by" date for thirty days. When I make chicken soup, I freeze the extra broth and use it for gravy for roast chicken or Cornish game hen.

As a rule of thumb, homemade food is cheaper and of better quality than what one can buy commercially. There is an added bonus: One knows what is in the food.

Another virtue of a great sauce: Food freezes better in a sauce. My technique: Freeze the food with the sauce without puréeing it. Before serving, defrost and purée. Freezing the food in an unpuréed state maintains more flavor. (Sometimes it is more convenient to purée several servings at the same time and then freeze the puréed dish. Do what works for you in the purée kitchen.)

Instant thickeners are important for two reasons: the safety of the swallow, and the binding and stabilizing of the purée so that the components do not separate. See Resource Section for details.

One final hint: Patients with swallowing difficulties cannot eat very cold or very hot foods. I usually serve food that is heated to warm for 30 seconds in the microwave at 50 % power. Warm food is more comforting and satisfying than food at room temperature.

The Recipes

This cookbook represents the marriage of art and science: the art of great food meeting the science of purée.

Three themes inform these recipes. The first is clean eating: low fat, low salt, low sugar, fresh fruit and vegetables, and lean protein. The second theme is variety. The third is taste appeal, which is achieved through the use of healthy sauces and gravies.

Life is pressured these days, everyone is busy, especially the home cook. When you make it at home, even though it takes time, you do yourself and your patient a huge favor. You know what is in the food.

Like many of the best television chefs, I include convenience foods of high quality, without horrific ingredients such as high fructose corn syrup and refined sugars, without preservatives and additives. To make salmon in puff pastry, I use store-bought puff pastry.

I use frozen chopped spinach as a substitute for fresh spinach. Substitutions in these recipes to suit your own palate and that of your family are fine. Improvisation is fine. Use what is at hand.

Entrees

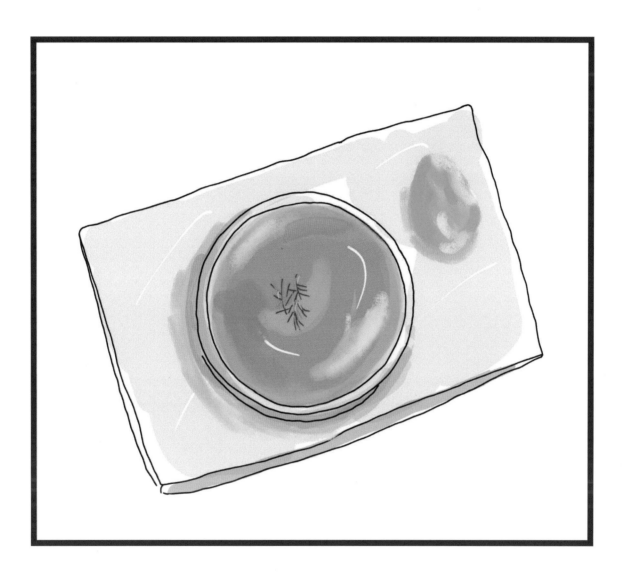

Chicken Pot Pie (Quickie Version)

PER SERVING

Calories	261
Fat	6 g.
Saturated Fat	1 g.
Sodium	181 mg.
Sugar	3 g,
Carbohydrate	46 g.
Fiber	9 g.
Protein	9 g.

Prep Time: 20 minutes
Cook Time: 8 to 15 minutes
Level: Medium
Serves 4

Ingredients

- Two chicken breasts, 1 lb., from store bought rotisserie chicken, cut into half inch cubes You can use dark meat if you prefer. Each pie has 4 oz. of chicken.
- One medium carrot, pan sautéed until medium soft or steamed soft, sliced into a small dice. (alternatively, use frozen diced carrots)
- ½ to 1 cup frozen peas, depending on how much you like peas
- Cream of chicken soup, I use health food store variety or supermarket variety with minimum preservatives, thinned with half the amount of liquid called for. Possible to use cream of mushroom or cream of celery.
- Store bought pie crust (can be whole grain), room temperature
- 1 egg lightly beaten with 1 tbsp. water, for egg wash
- Instant thickener

Directions

This is a deconstructed chicken pot pie. The filling is made separately from the crust. The same technique may be used for all the varieties of pot pie to follow.

For The Crust

Preheat the oven to 400 degrees.

Prepare a baking sheet with parchment paper or a silicone baking mat so the crusts won't stick.

On a board, open up the crust. Using a five inch bowl, cut two rounds of pie crust.

Mix an egg with 2 tablespoons of water and brush the surface of the crust with egg wash so it will brown.

Place the sheet pan in the oven.

When the crusts are golden, about eight minutes, remove and allow to cool.

For the Filling

Place condensed chicken soup in a saucepan over low heat. Whisk in liquid, milk or water, half the amount called for in package directions.

Add cooked chicken, carrots and peas. If using frozen carrots, place them in liquid first and allow them to cook three minutes until tender. Small diced carrots from frozen would be best for purée. If using cooked carrots, add all ingredients at the same time.

Allow to simmer gently for three or four minutes until ingredients are warmed through.

This is your filling. You now have filling and crust.

For the Purée

Take the two cooled crusts and break into the bowl of a mini food processor. Soften with two tablespoons warm broth or warm water.

Pulse to break up. Purée until smooth. Add a pump or a scoop of instant thickener. Purée 10 seconds to combine.

Place puréed crusts into a glass storage bowl. Cover. Place in fridge to set up good purée texture.

Clean bowl of food processor. Place 1 cup of filling in the bowl of the mini food processor. Pulse five times to break up the chicken. Purée until smooth. Add a pump or a scoop of instant thickener to thicken.

Divide filling between two glass storage bowls.

Spoon half of the crust onto each bowl of filling.

You now have two virtual reality puréed chicken pot pies composed of a layer of filling topped by a layer of crust.

Use this same method of puréeing for all pot pie recipes that follow.

Label the lids with the name of the dish, the date prepared and a "Use By" date (see Food Storage section). Place the pot pies in the fridge or in the freezer.

Equipment: Eventually you may want to acquire a second mini food processor. Many recipes have two main ingredients. Using a processor for a crust or a topping, or a protein, with a second processor for the second component of the dish, cuts down prep time. The cleaning of the bowl of a second food processor requires minimal labor. You could also use a combination of the mini food processor for the crust and the small pitcher of a Ninja for the filling.

Purée 1 cup of filling at a time until smooth. Thicken with one pump of thickener.

Divide filling into two 4 ½ inch glass storage bowls. (Thickened items stick to plastic containers),

Spoon thickened crust on top.

You now have a two-layer puréed chicken pot pie.

To Serve

Warm in a microwave at 50% power for 30 seconds. If necessary, add time in increments of 10 seconds to warm the pie. If pie is frozen, thaw in fridge for two hours.

Chicken Pot Pie (From Scratch)

Serves 4

Ingredients

- 1 lb. chicken breasts, skinless and boneless, cut into half inch cubes
- 1 carrot, cut into small dice
- 1 cup frozen peas
- Store bought pie crust
- Four individual dishes, I use bowls that are oven safe, such as Le Creuset or any good stoneware
- One half sheet pan for putting the bowls in the oven to bake
- 2 cups chicken stock, either store bought or homemade
- 2 tbsp. flour, unbleached whole wheat pastry flour is my choice
- Instant thickener

Directions

Preheat oven to 400 degrees.

For the Crust

Line a baking sheet with parchment paper or a silicone liner. Cut two circles of pie crust or puff pastry the size of a four and a half inch glass storage bowl. Trace around the bowl with a knife, using the dish as a stencil.

Place the rounds of pie crust on the baking sheet and brush with an egg wash made of an egg lightly beaten with water. You may also use cream to paint the crust.

Place the sheet in the oven and bake for twelve minutes for the puff pastry or eight minutes for the pie crust.

Remove the sheet pan from the oven and place on a trivet and allow to cool.

This is your deconstructed crust.

For the Filling

Use 2 tbsp. of oil, I use canola or extra virgin olive oil. I use cold pressed oils. Warm in a sauce pan. Add 2 tbsp. flour and cook for a minute until flour is no longer raw.

Warm 2 cups stock so that you are not adding cold liquid to the roux. Stir into the roux a little at a time, say a quarter of a cup at a time, once the flour is dissolved. One does not want lumps. OK to use a whisk. If you use the entire two cups of flour, you will have a thin sauce. If you like a thick sauce, use 1 ½ cups stock.

I use an electric wok to stir fry the chicken. I add two tbsp. of peanut oil or any oil that does not have a strong flavor, such as canola oil or grapeseed oil. I turn the wok to high and sear the chicken for approximately five minutes or until it is golden. I add the diced carrots and peas and I add the thickened broth. If you are not using an electric wok or fry pan, use a plain skillet, larger size to accommodate the filling.

Assemble the pot pie by filling each dish with one quarter of the filling, then place the pie crust on top, rolling it onto a rolling pin or gently lifting it with a long spatula.

Crimp the edges of the top over the sides of the dish. Brush with egg wash and cut two steam holes of about a half inch in the top of the crust.

Then purée. For freezing, I wrap the pie in the dish in clear wrap, then in foil, then enclose in a lock and store dish and note that it should be used within two weeks.

Tip: You can add any other vegetable, such as frozen pearl onions. Change the traditional carrots and peas for sautéed mushrooms and cream of mushroom soup.

A Shortcut

For the time-challenged cook, how to deconstruct a pot pie for the dysphagia kitchen:

When you get the filling in the wok or the sautée pan, cook it until the chicken is done, approximately seven minutes at a low simmer. Cut the rounds of the pie crust to size and put them on the baking sheet lined with parchment paper. Bake in the oven according to package directions for a one-crust pie. This is about twelve minutes for puff pastry and a little shorter for pie crust. This will be puréed, so the beauty of presentation is not as important as the taste of the final pot pie.

For the Purée

Break up a crust into the bowl of a mini food processor and soften with two or three tablespoons of warm broth or water. Add instant thickener. Purée.

Place crust in a glass storage bowl, cover, and place in the fridge to set up.

Rinse out the mini food processor and blade. Add 3/4 cup of filling to the mini food processor. Pulse to break up and then purée. Add instant thickener.

Place puréed filling in a glass bowl. Top with puréed crust.

You now have a puréed chicken pot pie. There should be twice as much filling in the bowl as crust, just as in a real world pie.

Please make sure that both the filling and the crust are the same thickness for the swallow.

If your kitchen is equipped with two mini food processors, use one for the crust and one for the filling. This cuts down on prep time.

To Serve

Warm at 50% power in the microwave for twenty seconds to serve warm.

Seafood Pot Pie (From Scratch)

Serves 4

PER SERVING

Calories	199
Fat	10 g.
Saturated Fat	2 g.
Sodium	331 mg.
Sugar	1 g.
Carbohydrate	11 g.
Fiber	2 g.
Protein	18 g.

Ingredients

- 2 lobster tails steamed with lemon juice and tarragon in steaming liquid. Or 8 marinated and sautéed sea scallops or a combination of 4 marinated scallops plus 8 cooked shrimp. You can use lobster bisque (Bar Harbor brand available in supermarket, at desired thickness) or a cream of shrimp soup for liquid
- Seafood stock for thickened broth as prepared above for chicken pot pie
- 1 bunch baby spinach, wilted
- 1 tablespoon olive oil
- 1 teaspoon lemon juice
- 1 small shallot, sliced thinly (optional)
- 1 clove garlic, sliced thinly (optional)
- Pie crust or puff pastry, store bought, at room temperature.

Directions

Lobster Pot Pie is a festive pot pie that I make on New Years' Day.

Steam the lobster tail until the shell is red and the meat is still soft. Don't dry out the meat by overcooking. Alternatively, you can broil the tail or grill it. I paint the shell with olive oil. Remove meat from shell. Cut into inch cubes. I use one 6 oz. tail per pie.

Wilt the spinach with a little olive oil and some thinly slices shallot and garlic, if desired.

Assemble the filling in the same way. Warm up the lobster bisque in a saucepan. Place wilted spinach and lobster in filling until warm. Do not overcook steamed lobster. Keep the protein tender by not overcooking. Biggest danger with seafood is that when it is overcooked, it gets rubbery. Not good for the purée or for the swallow.

If you are making a thickened seafood broth, follow the directions as above for a thickened chicken stock, substituting seafood stock, or even lobster stock. I save my lobster shells and freeze them, and then when I have enough, I make a lobster stock by cooking them for fifteen minutes in three quarts of water with an onion and a carrot.

For the Crust

Line a baking sheet with parchment paper or a silicone liner. Cut two circles of pie crust or puff pastry the size of a four and a half inch glass storage bowl. Trace around the bowl with a knife, using the dish as a stencil.

Place the rounds of pie crust on the baking sheet and brush with an egg wash made of an egg lightly beaten with water. You may also use cream to paint the crust.

Place the sheet in the oven and bake for twelve minutes for the puff pastry or eight minutes for the pie crust.

Remove the sheet pan from the oven and place on a trivet and allow to cool.

This is your deconstructed crust.

For the Purée

Break up a crust into the bowl of a mini food processor and soften with two or three tablespoons of warm broth or water. Add instant thickener. Purée.

Add to the bottom of a glass storage bowl, about ¼ in thick. This will taste like pie crust, but will be in a puréed form. To the eye, there will be a separation between the crust and the filling.

Cover the bowl and allow to set in the refrigerator while you purée the filling.

Rinse out the mini food processor and blade. Add 3/4 cup of filling to the mini food processor. Pulse to break up and then purée. Add instant thickener.

Add filling to the bowl with the crust.

Warm at 50% power in the microwave for twenty seconds to serve warm. The spoon goes down through the filling to get a third of a spoon of crust on the spoon. Please make sure that both the filling and the crust are the same thickness for the swallow.

If your kitchen is equipped with two mini food processors, use one for the crust and one for the filling. This cuts down on prep time.

Scallop and Shrimp Pot Pie

Most scallops are flash-frozen on the boat upon harvesting. I thaw mine out in room temperature water in a bowl in the refrigerator. I pat them dry and marinate them in a two tablespoons vegetable oil, a tablespoon of lemon juice and a little Old Bay seasoning. May add garlic if desired.

For an Asian hot and sour marinade, use 2 tablespoons peanut oil or vegetable oil, 2 tablespoons rice wine vinegar, a teaspoon of dark sesame oil, and two dashes soy sauce.

You can buy fresh shrimp and stir fry them in a little oil until pink. For a quickie pot pie, you can buy frozen cooked tail on shrimp and thaw them in cool water in a bowl in the fridge. Then assemble.

For the Crust

Line a baking sheet with parchment paper or a silicone liner. Cut two circles of pie crust or puff pastry the size of a four and a half inch glass storage bowl. Trace around the bowl with a knife, using the dish as a stencil.

Place the rounds of pie crust on the baking sheet and brush with an egg wash made of an egg lightly beaten with water. You may also use cream to paint the crust.

Place the sheet in the oven and bake for twelve minutes for the puff pastry or eight minutes for the pie crust.

Remove the sheet pan from the oven and place on a trivet and allow to cool.

This is your deconstructed crust.

For the Purée

Take one of the cooled crusts and break it into the bowl of a mini food processor.

Soften with two tablespoons warm broth or warm water.

Pulse to break up. Purée. Add a tablespoon of instant thickener, powder or gel. Purée.

Add to a glass storage bowl that has a lid, Pyrex or Anchor Hocking, four and a half inches.

Place crust in fridge to set.

Clean bowl of food processor.

Purée 3/4 cup of filling. Thicken.

Add to the bowl. Cover.

Warm in a microwave at 50% power for 30 seconds. Serve.

Vegetable Pot Pies

Serves 4

PER SERVING

Calories	159
Fat	11 g.
Saturated Fat	2 g.
Sodium	522 mg.
Sugar	1 g.
Carbohydrate	14 g.
Fiber	2 g.
Protein	3 g.

The method of purée is the same as for the chicken pot pie.

Broccoli and Cheddar Pot Pie

- 2 cups lightly steamed broccoli florets cut into bite size pieces
- Cheddar Soup, blended with half the amount of liquid or thickened as the base

Lightly steam the broccoli and add to cheddar soup.
Use this as the filling and prepare in the same manner as the chicken pot pie.

Asparagus And Mushroom Pot Pie

- Steamed asparagus and cream of mushroom soup as the filling.
- 1 bunch of asparagus, steamed, and cut into bite size pieces or frozen asparagus tips.

Prep is the same as for the chicken pot pie. Lightly steam the asparagus and add to thickened mushroom soup as the filling. Add ¼ cup grated Monterey Jack cheese for protein.

Mushroom Pot Pie

Mushroom Pot Pie uses a variety of mushrooms, such as shiitake, baby bella and white button and any other mushroom, such as the oyster mushroom. Select a variety of what is available in the market. Lightly sauté with a shot of soy sauce, garlic and thyme, and use in a cream of mushroom soup base. Add ¼ cup grated Gruyère cheese for protein.

Vegetable Ragout Pot Pie

One may vary the vegetables according to individual taste or even use leftovers of grilled or steamed or roasted vegetables. Use mixed vegetables can contain broccoli, cauliflower, zucchini, string beans, Brussel sprouts, and even lightly steamed squash such as butternut squash for sweetness.

You can go with a straight cream of asparagus soup or cream of celery soup for the base or one can make a curried veggie pot pie. You can use butternut squash soup or even red pepper soup as the base. For variety, one can use a small amount of curry sauce in coconut milk as the base. Add ¼ cup grated parmesan or cheddar or goat cheese. These are easy and quick and infinitely better than anything commercially packaged.

Beef Pot Pie

Serves 4

Calories	173
Fat	8 g.
Saturated Fat	3 g.
Sodium	56 mg.
Sugar	4 g.
Carbohydrate	14 g.
Fiber	2 g.
Protein	11 g.

Ingredients

- 6 oz. leftover pot roast with gravy and vegetables. Cut pot roast into inch cubes.

Directions

Heat up filling and prepare puff pastry tops in oven, covered with egg wash, cooked about twelve minutes, according to instructions on package. Assemble pie in dish by adding filling and top.

Purée, adding extra stock or gravy as needed.

For the Crust

Line a baking sheet with parchment paper or a silicone liner. Cut two circles of pie crust or puff pastry the size of a four

and a half inch glass storage bowl. Trace around the bowl with a knife, using the dish as a stencil.

Place the rounds of pie crust on the baking sheet and brush with an egg wash made of an egg lightly beaten with water. You may also use cream to paint the crust.

Place the sheet in the oven and bake for twelve minutes for the puff pastry or eight minutes for the pie crust.

Remove the sheet pan from the oven and place on a trivet and allow to cool.

This is your deconstructed crust.

For the Purée

Break up a crust into the bowl of a mini food processor and soften with two or three tablespoons of warm broth or water. Add instant thickener. Purée.

Add to the bottom of a glass storage bowl, about ¼ in thick. This will taste like pie crust, but will be in a puréed form.

To the eye, there will be a separation between the crust and the filling.

Cover the bowl and allow to set in the refrigerator while you purée the filling.

Rinse out the mini food processor and blade. Add 3/4 cup of filling to the mini food processor. Pulse to break up and then purée. Add instant thickener.

Add filling to the bowl with the crust.

Warm at 50% power in the microwave for twenty seconds to serve warm. The spoon goes down through the filling to get a third of a spoon of crust on the spoon. Please make sure that both the filling and the crust are the same thickness for the swallow.

If your kitchen is equipped with two mini food processors, use one for the crust and one for the filling. This cuts down on prep time.

Beef Stew

Prep Time: 15 minutes
Cook Time: 2 hours
Level: Easy
Serves 6

Calories	353
Fat	13 g.
Saturated Fat	5 g.
Sodium	473 mg.
Sugar	4 g.
Carbohydrate	22 g.
Fiber	4 g.
Protein	36 g.

Ingredients

- 2 lbs. stewing beef, trimmed of extra fat and silver skin
- 1 medium onion, diced
- 1 clove garlic, minced
- 2 carrots, halved and sliced into half moon slices
- Chicken or beef stock, 1 quart, may be homemade or store bought, lower sodium variety.
- 1 tbsp. tomato paste thinned with 3 tbsps. water
- Shot of lower sodium soy sauce
- 1 pound potatoes, peeled and cubed into one inch cubes
- Half package of frozen peas

Directions

Remove all silver skin and excess fat from beef with a good paring knife. Season with salt and white pepper. Brown in 2 tbsp. vegetable oil. Set aside.

Brown onions, add carrot, and at the end, add the garlic. Mix the tomato paste with the water and soy sauce and brown with the veggies.

Add the beef back in to either a dutch oven. Add peeled and cubed potatoes. Add chicken stock or just plain water to cover ingredients.

Bring to boil. Cook for two hours on low. May also be cooked in a slow cooker on low for four hours. This is a braising technique that is used with less expensive cuts of meat, often the most flavorful, that renders them tender and delicious.

At the end, add the peas. (These have already been steamed before freezing, so can be added without cooking in advance.)

This purées very nicely and also freezes nicely.

Veal Stew: Buy the veal stewing meat in the grocery store and trim it of all silver skin and extra fat. The silver skin becomes very tough and chewy when cooked. When making veal stew, I substitute sweet potato for white potato. Follow directions for lamb stew. Use 2 lbs. of veal.

Lamb Stew: I also make lamb stew, using lamb shoulder, trimmed down. Use 2 pounds of lamb shoulder, cut into inch and a half cubes.

Directions for Veal or Lamb

Season either veal or lamb with salt and white pepper, and brown in olive oil.

Remove from pan. Cook onion and carrot. Whisk in half a small can of tomato paste, thinned and whisked with a quarter cup of water. Brown the tomato paste in with the vegetables to develop its flavor.

Add veal or lamb back in. Add a half cup of red wine if your patient can tolerate it. Also add a sprig of fresh rosemary. Add four cups of chicken broth.

Peel one large or two medium sweet potatoes into inch cubes. Cook them for two hours along with the stew.

Use a slurry of a tablespoon of flour mixed with water to thin consistency, to thicken the gravy, bringing to the boil gently and slowly simmering for five minutes until the raw taste of the flour goes away.

Shepherd's Pie

If you have leftover lamb stew, put it in a baking dish and cover with a recipe of homemade mashed potato. Place mashed potatoes over lamb stew and dot with butter or non trans-fat margarine. Place in 350 degree oven and bake for fifteen minutes until the potatoes are browned a little on top. Makes an excellent purée.

For the Purée

When the dish is cooled, add 1 cup of the dish to the bowl of a mini food processor.

Pulse five times to break down the elements of the dish.

Then purée until smooth.

If the dish is too thick, add gravy or broth.

If the dish is too thin, add potatoes or instant thickener until the correct thickness is reached.

 Tip: When in need of a quick recipe of mashed potatoes, try Edward & Sons Organic Mashed Potatoes. Ready in five minutes. Superior to supermarket brands. No chemicals or preservatives. Clean eating.

Pot Roast

Calories	392
Fat	17 g.
Saturated Fat	6 g.
Sodium	496 mg.
Sugar	3 g.
Carbohydrate	15 g.
Fiber	3 g.
Protein	43 g.

Prep Time: 15 minutes
Cook Time: 4 hours slow cooker
Level: Easy
Serves 6

Ingredients

- 2½ pounds beef shoulder or chuck roast
- 1 large yellow onion, diced
- 3 carrots, peeled and cut into sections
- 1 container chicken broth or one quart chicken broth (use beef broth if you prefer)
- Olive oil
- Salt and white pepper
- A shot of lower sodium soy sauce
- One pound potatoes, cut into large cubes

Directions

Trim fat and remove silver skin from beef, liberally season the beef on both sides and brown in olive oil in a skillet until you have a sear on both sides. Remove and put on platter and cover with foil to keep warm.

Sauté the onion in a little olive oil, add carrots and sauté for two minutes.

Put all ingredients in a slow cooker and cook for four hours. I use the lower sodium soy sauce to add depth of flavor to my sauce.

I boil my potatoes separately in salted water for 20 minutes until fork tender. I do this to make sure they are exactly the right consistency.

Alternatively, you can place the meat and vegetables and broth in a Dutch oven in a 350 degree oven and cook for two hours. You can add the potatoes for the last hour.

When roast is done, it will fall apart. Remove all ingredients from the cooker or Dutch oven, except for the broth. Using 2 tsp. of flour whisked into 2 tsp. of water, create a slurry and pour into the broth, stirring. Bring to a boil and simmer for three minutes, until the raw flavor of the flour is gone and the broth thickens to the desired consistency.

For the Purée

After the dish has cooled, place one cup of the dish in the bowl of a mini food processor or the pitcher of a flat bottomed blender, such as the Ninja.

Pulse five times to break down the elements of the dish.

Purée until smooth.

Use potato to thicken the dish. Use instant thickener if necessary.

This freezes beautifully in individual portions. Make sure you have enough of the sauce. Make sure you leave a third of the freezer safe storage dish empty. Liquids expand when freezing.

Eggplant Parmesan Light

Calories	245
Fat	11 g.
Saturated Fat	5 g.
Sodium	201 mg.
Sugar	7 g.
Carbohydrate	25 g.
Fiber	10 g.
Protein	16 g.

Prep Time: 30 minutes
Cook Time: 45 minutes
Level: Intermediate
Serves 6

This is a French version of the dish that does not require breading and deep frying. I make it using extra virgin olive oil about an eighth of an inch deep. Heat the pan and when the oil is hot, drop in the eggplant slices. If the oil level goes down for the second side of the eggplant, I use lower sodium chicken broth. This keeps the oil content down and also adds excellent flavor to the dish. Vegetable broth could be used as well. I have doctored and adapted the basic idea which is from The Barefoot Contessa.

Ingredients

- One medium eggplant. Pick a good shape that will give even slices for your baking pan. Use a knife to get the slices even or a mandolin.
- Extra virgin olive oil for sauté
- Lower sodium chicken broth for sauté
- One jar favorite pasta sauce. I use Florentine, for the spinach. Homemade is always good if you make a big pot, a gallon, and then store in quart containers in freezer.

If desired, meat to add protein to dish. I use either chicken sausage or ground turkey with plenty of fresh herbs added: parsley, oregano, basil, the classics in whatever proportion you like.

Topping

- 2 cups part skim milk ricotta
- ¼ cup grated parmesan cheese
- 2 extra large eggs
- Freshly chopped parsley, one tablespoon
- Freshly chopped basil, one tablespoon
- Salt and white pepper to taste, about a half teaspoon salt and a quarter teaspoon pepper.

Prep

Brown sausage or ground meat in pan with a small amount of oil

Slice eggplant approximately 3/8 inch thick

Put a quarter inch of olive oil in fry pan and heat until rippling

Cook eggplant until it begins to soften on the first side, and flip. Approximately two to three minutes a side.

Remove eggplant to plate with paper towel for draining and add salt and white pepper

Proceed until all eggplant is cooked.

Filling

Mix ricotta and parmesan, herbs, salt and white pepper, with the two eggs, lightly beaten. Add a tablespoon or two of milk if texture is not smooth and creamy. Mixture should be loose. Mozzarella should be the fresh variety or eliminate it altogether, for ease of swallowing.

Assembly

To the bottom of a 9 x 13 baking dish, add a cup of pasta sauce and smooth it over the bottom of the dish. This prevents sticking.

Place a single layer of the cooked eggplant and cover with the remainder of your sauce.

Top with filling, sprinkle with additional parmesan.

Bake in 375 degree oven for 35 minutes, until bubbling. Carefully remove from oven and let cool and set before serving.

For the Purée

The purée for this dish is very simple because it has a sauce. Because of the ricotta cheese mixture, one serving approximately four inches square will have a larger volume than it appears on the plate. This is normal. The dish is very light and airy in purée.

Use instant thickener if necessary to stabilize the purée so that sauce does not separate.

Stuffed Shells and Oven Roasted Turkey Meatballs

PER SERVING

Calories	336
Fat	13 g.
Saturated Fat	8 g.
Sodium	320 mg
Sugar	7 g.
Carbohydrate	31 g.
Fiber	3 g.
Protein	19 g.

Prep Time: 15 Minutes
Cook Time: 30 minutes
Level: Easy
Serves 4

Ingredients

- 9 jumbo shells
- 1 jar of pasta sauce
- Parmigiano reggiano cheese

Filling

- 2 cups ricotta cheese, part skim if cholesterol is an issue
- ⅓ cup Parmigiano reggiano
- 1 egg
- Salt and white pepper
- 2 tbsp. Italian parsley, chopped finely

Directions

Preheat oven to 350 degrees.

In four quarts of salted water, boil shells according to package directions, cooking them half way.

In an 8 x 8 baking dish, add the pasta sauce, doctoring it in any way you like, by adding sautéed sausage (I use the chicken sausage from the Greenway section of the Publix market. (The chicken is raised without antibiotics and is additive and preservative free) or ground meat, or sautéed mushrooms and a clove or two of garlic sliced thinly and sautéed for a minute in olive oil, or add a handful of finely chopped fresh basil from the herb garden.

Prepare filling by mixing ricotta cheese, Parmigiano and beaten egg with salt and white pepper and parsley. Using a tablespoon, fill the shells.

Line up shells in sauce, spacing them evenly. Cover with foil. Bake in 350 degree oven for thirty-five minutes until bubbling. Allow to cool.

For the Purée

Place two or three stuffed shells in the bowl of a mini food processor or the pitcher of a blender. Add 1/3 cup sauce.

If desired, break up two turkey meatballs in the food processor or blender.

Pulse five times to break up ingredients and blend with sauce.

Purée until smooth.

Instant thickener may be added to stabilize the purée. Use one pump or one scoop.

Diane's Turkey Meatballs

Prep Time: 10 minutes
Cook Time: 42 minutes
Level: Medium
Serves 8

PER SERVING

Calories	120
Fat	5 g.
Saturated Fat	2 g.
Sodium	203 mg
Sugar	0 g.
Carbohydrate	5 g.
Fiber	0 g.
Protein	12 g.

Ingredients

- 1 package ground turkey, 1 lb.
- 1 extra large egg
- 2 tbsp. grated Parmigiano reggiano or Romano cheese
- 2 tbsp. flat leaf parsley chopped fine
- Salt and white pepper
- 1 garlic clove, grated using a hand grater
- ¼ cup bread crumbs, Italian seasoned or homemade from day old baguette
- A shake of extra virgin olive oil for moisture and richness

Directions

Preheat oven to 425 degrees. Prepare half baking sheet with rack.

In a bowl, mix the ground turkey, the beaten egg, the cheese, the parsley, garlic, salt and white pepper and enough crumbs to make a mixture that is not too wet and not too dry, about a third of a cup. Mix lightly and do not overwork. You can chill the mixture if it makes it easier to work. If forming meatballs with your hands, keep your hands damp for ease of handling and also do not pack your meatballs tight but gently press them together. Sometimes I add a teaspoon of olive oil to the mixture just to enrich the taste. Turkey has almost no fat and a little fat makes the meatballs taste delicious.

Using a small ice cream scoop, make one-inch meat balls and place on rack. Do not pack tightly. Gently form the meatball. (Use pastry brush, paint with olive oil.)

Flash roast in oven for fifteen minutes on 425 degrees until meat ball browns on all sides. This is the purpose of the rack. This eliminates the step where you brown the meatballs in a pan of oil, which is messy and adds a lot of oil to the dish.

When meatballs have a brown crust, remove sheet from oven and put meatballs into a pot containing about a quart of sauce, whether store bought or your own.

Cook for about twenty minutes in the sauce at a simmer. The meatballs will flavor the sauce and the sauce provides you with your purée medium. Makes 16 meatballs.

For the Purée

When meatballs cool, break up three or four in the bowl of a mini food processor or the pitcher of a blender.

Add one half cup sauce.

Pulse five times to break down meatballs.

Purée until smooth.

May be served as a snack by themselves.

May be added to the stuffed shells dish. See directions above.

Tip: Ground beef may be used for meatballs if this is the flavor profile that seems best in your care plan. You can mix beef with pork or veal, ½ pound each.

Tip: Keep turkey chilled and work quickly. Egg should be at room temperature, beaten lightly. The mixture forms balls nicely. The secret to a tender meatball is not to pack the meat too tightly. If mixture is too wet to form meatballs nicely, add a little more bread crumb.

Tip: Freeze the extra meatballs, 4 to a container along with a cup of sauce. This will come in handy for a quick dinner. Boil pasta for two servings. Add meatballs and sauce, four meatballs, one cup sauce and two servings pasta for two dinners. I usually purée right before serving for best flavor. One meal is served. One goes in the fridge for later in the week. Or goes into the freezer. The stored meals are only puréed when it is time to serve them.

Stuffed Peppers

Prep Time: 20 minutes
Cook Time: 1 hour
Level: Intermediate
Serves 4

PER SERVING

Calories	253
Fat	5 g.
Saturated Fat	1 g.
Sodium	48 mg.
Sugar	6 g.
Carbohydrate	38 g.
Fiber	3 g.
Protein	14 g.

This was a great favorite of my mother's. One is served on the day of its preparation. One goes into the fridge for serving two or three days later. Two go into the freezer in individual portions, labeled with the date of creation and the USE BY date.

Green peppers do not agree with my mom, so I use red, yellow and orange. Please feel free to use your favorite pepper.

For variation, I use different grains. I use brown basmati rice, barley, fine grain kasha and quinoa. Quinoa should be rinsed before cooking.

Prepare the grains according to the instructions in the Whole Grains section, using either a rice cooker or an electric pressure cooker. This is to completely soften the grain for the smooth purée and the safety of the swallow. The rice cooker will set its own cooking cycle. The electric pressure cooker will take up to 40 minutes

Please use any type of protein. I have used ground beef, ground turkey, ground chicken, ground lamb, and the insides of organic sausage made from either turkey or pork. For a vegetarian version, use tofu or tempeh sausage purchased in the whole foods store. I usually do not prepare this dish with seafood, but there is no reason the peppers could not be stuffed with shrimp. In this case, I would pre-cook the peppers in the sauce until almost soft, since the shrimp require a short oven time, four or five minutes, until opaque.

Ingredients
- 2 medium red peppers

Filling
- Two cups cooked rice or quinoa or buckwheat groats
- 1 shallot sautéed (may be red, yellow, white or green onion)
- 1 clove minced garlic

- 1 cup chicken sausage meat, browned. May be any other type of meat.

Filling Directions

Sauté shallot and garlic, add cooked rice, stir to incorporate.

I use a dash of soy sauce (lower sodium) and add herbs, dried or fresh parsley, minced.

Add browned sausage meat and incorporate.

Sauce

- 1 can diced tomatoes, plain or flavored with garlic, basil, 15 oz.
- 1 small can tomato sauce *If you choose, you can substitute a container of tomato bisque*

Directions

The idea is to make the rice filling have a soft creamy texture like that of risotto. This makes for a wonderful purée texture.

Cut red peppers in half lengthwise. The traditional presentation for stuffed peppers is to cut off the top and bake standing up. This is difficult for purée, so I have adopted the lengthwise cut.

Fill each half of the pepper with the filling, mounting it up. Approximately ¾ cup.

Place filled peppers in a 9 x 9 baking dish. Add diced tomatoes and sauce or bisque slightly more than halfway up the side of the pepper.

Cover with aluminum foil. Bake at 350 degrees for an hour until pepper is soft.
This should give enough sauce to purée each serving. I then use one serving right away and put one serving the fridge for use during the week. USE BY date for all entrees stored in fridge is 1 week, with the exception of cooked seafood which is three days.

For the Purée

When the dish has cooled take one half a pepper for a small serving and two halves for a larger appetite.

Cut the peppers in half and add to the bowl of a mini food processor or the pitcher of a blender with a half cup of sauce. Pulse 10 times to break down ingredients, then purée until smooth.

Add sauce as necessary.

Rock Cornish Game Hens with Pan Gravy

PER SERVING

Calories	173
Fat	4 g.
Saturated Fat	1 g.
Sodium	243 mg.
Sugar	3 g.
Carbohydrate	8 g.
Fiber	2 g.
Protein	26 g.

Prep Time: 20 minutes
Cook Time: One hour
Level: Intermediate
Serves 4

These little hens have plenty of flavor and make enough food for two dinners and a small amount of chicken salad. A change from the normal roast chicken, although the recipe can be used for a roast chicken. If available, please buy the little hens that have never been frozen. Otherwise, thaw the frozen ones in the fridge.

Ingredients

- 2 Rock Cornish game hens, never frozen
- 1 lemon
- 2 sprigs rosemary
- 2 cloves garlic
- Olive oil
- Salt and white pepper
- Rack to go in roasting pan

In the roasting pan

- One cup chicken stock
- ¼ cup white wine (optional)
- One medium yellow onion cut in eighths
- 2 carrots, cut in sections
- 1 stalk celery cut in sections
- 1 bay leaf
- Salt and white pepper
- Several sprigs fresh flat leaf parsley

Directions

Preheat the oven to 400 degrees.

Wash the little hens thoroughly and pat dry. My father used to kosher the inside of the hens by covering the inside with salt, letting it rest a few minutes and then rinsing it out.

Arrange all the pan gravy ingredients in the bottom of the roasting pan. After the chickens are roasted, this will become your gravy. If there are giblets inside the little hens, take them out of their packages, rinse them, and put them in the chicken stock for flavoring.

Prepping the hens for roasting

Cut the lemon in half and insert half a lemon in the cavity of each bird. Add a sprig of rosemary and a clove of garlic inside the cavity of each bird. Rub the outside of the bird with olive oil, salt and white pepper. Put them on the rack next to each other, but not so close as to prevent circulation of air.

Roast in oven for twenty minutes to the pound. If bird is two pounds, forty minutes. Until juices run clear when one inserts a knife into the joint between the breast and the thigh.

Remove from oven and let clear.

For gravy, remove vegetables, herbs and giblets from pan. Vegetables may be eaten or puréed with gravy for thickness, excluding the celery, which can be stringy. If you like liver, the liver of the bird may also go right into the purée. Otherwise, discard the flavor elements. Make a slurry of two tablespoons of Wondraflour and two or three tablespoons of water, Put the roasting pan on a low heat, and add slurry to pan drippings, stirring slowly until mixture comes to a boil and thickens. Cook for five minutes at a simmer until the raw flavor of the flour disappears.

For the Purée

When the bird has cooled, take four to six ounces of meat and break it off the bird. Place in the bowl of a mini food processor or in the small pitcher of a blender. Add a half cup of gravy.

Pulse 10 times to break up the protein, then purée until smooth. Add instant thickener if necessary to get the desired thickness. If desired, add a half cup of softly cooked rice and more gravy for the purée.

The side dish can be mashed sweet potato. See recipe. Can also be served with a side vegetable.

For service, I use separate plates with separate colors of food, the eating with the eyes principal.

Cornish Hen Salad

Serves 2

Calories	224
Fat	11 g.
Saturated Fat	3 g.
Sodium	210 mg.
Sugar	1 g.
Carbohydrate	3 g.
Fiber	0 g.
Protein	26 g.

As I mentioned before, I try not to waste food. Here's a good meal made from the leftovers of the Cornish game hen recipe.

For the Purée

Take the leftover roasted meat, wings and legs, and add to a food processor or the small pitcher of a blender.

Add 1 tablespoon of your favorite mayonnaise and 1 tablespoon of lower fat sour cream and 1 tablespoon of water. Salt and white pepper to taste.

Pulse five times to blend ingredients and break them down. Purée. This gives a creamy loose hen salad of the classic American variety. Add a little chopped flat leaf parsley for color.

If extra liquid is needed, use water. Don't water down the flavors with too much water. Chicken stock may be used.

Keep stock refrigerated for food safety.

For service, place a cup of the chicken salad in a bowl.

Beef, Shrimp, Lobster, Lamb, or Vegetable Curry

PER SERVING

Calories	285
Fat	15 g.
Saturated Fat	5 g.
Sodium	568 mg.
Sugar	2 g.
Carbohydrate	13 g.
Fiber	2 g.
Protein	25 g.

Prep Time: 10 minutes
Cook Time: 10 minutes
Level: Easy
Serves 2

A very mild curry, thinned with coconut milk or yogurt, is a flavorful sauce, perfect for purée. Make sure you get clearance from your healthcare provider. There are many different varieties of curry, from Indian to Thai and various curries of the Caribbean. The reason that I make curry is quite simply the flavor.

Starting an Indian curry from scratch is a process that takes a long time because of the blending of spices. So for Indian curry, I use a very good quality sauce that I buy in the whole foods store. It is one of my "go to" convenience ingredients. It is the Ethnic Gourmet, Calcutta Masala, which I buy because it is mild in flavor and easy on my mother's digestion. There are several other curry choices in this brand. A new discovery is the Royal Curry Delight brand of simmer sauces.

A Thai curry is easier. Thai Kitchen now makes a Panang Curry Sauce that is available in the ethnic section of the supermarket. It is a simmer sauce, and one does not have to do any mixing.

Taste the sauce and see if it will work for the person with swallowing difficulty. You do not want heat. You do not want the person to cough or have a sharp intake of the breath.

Ingredients

- One good 8 oz. steak, sliced very thinly across the grain
- ½ jar Ethnic Gourmet Calcutta Masala Sauce
  Or Thai Kitchen Panang Curry Sauce or Royal Curry Delight simmer sauce, Tikka Masala variety

Directions

Season the steak slices lightly with salt and white pepper. Sear in a hot fry pan about a minute on each side

Add curry sauce and greens. This can be a cup of frozen spinach or kale or chard and cook for four minutes. In prepping the greens, remove veins and stems. For kale or chard, a quick three minute steam or sauté will render them tender and digestible. Use ¼ cup greens per serving. Add a half cup of cooked basmati rice and you have the purée.

Serving is one cup of beef with curry sauce, eyeballing about 4 oz. of the beef and about a half cup of the curry sauce, with the ¼ cup of greens and ½ cup of cooked rice.

VARIATIONS

To keep excitement about the food, vary the protein:

Chicken Curry

For chicken curry, substitute one pound of chicken breast cut into one-inch cubes.

Seafood Curry

A half pound of shrimp, tail on but shell split and deveined, for flavor. Heat 1 tbsp. of oil in pan and get some color on each side of the shrimp. Add the curry sauce and cook until shrimp turn bright pink. Remove shells when mixture is cool, before purée. Cooking the shrimp in the curry sauce with the shell on increases the flavor.

Or a couple of lobster tails. Same process. Add some oil in the pan and swirl the tails until they get a light sear. Add the curry sauce.

Lamb Curry

In one of the John Le Carré espionage novels, the author speaks of his hero seeing God after his first experience of eating lamb vindaloo. Lamb vindaloo is a hot curry, but you don't have to make it that hot.

Use a pound of lamb shoulder, cut into one inch cubes. Brown the cubes of lamb in a tablespoon of hot vegetable oil and then cook for some 10 minutes in the simmering curry sauce. You can add a little sour cream to make a creamy curry that resembles tikka masala.

Vegetable Curry

For a vegan version of this dish, one may purée firm tofu in the sauce. Silken tofu is too soft and gives a milkshake consistency of purée rather than a more substantial purée. Add one block of tofu, cut into 1 inch cubes and warmed through in the curry sauce, for the protein boost.

For the Purée

When the dish has cooled, in the bowl of a mini food processor or the small pitcher of a blender, place a cup of the curry with protein and sauce.

Serving should be 4 oz. of the protein, ¼ cup of greens, ½ cup of soft-cooked basmati rice. See the directions in the Whole Grains section.

Traditional accompaniments:

One may add a tablespoon of yogurt and a tablespoon of chutney as long as the chutney is sweet, not hot.

Pulse the dish about 10 times to incorporate all the elements. Purée until smooth.

Instant thickener may be added to stabilize the purée.

Roast Loin of Pork Three Ways

Prep Time: 10 minutes
Cook Time: 1 hour
Level: Easy
Serves 6

Ingredients

- 2 lbs. Loin of Pork
- 2 tbsp. vegetable oil
- Salt and white pepper
- Lower sodium soy sauce
- 2 cloves garlic, sliced thinly

Directions

Preheat oven to 350 degrees.

Make small slits in pork and insert slices of garlic.

Rub loin with 1 tbsp. oil and 1 tbsp. lower sodium soy sauce, salt and white pepper.

Use remaining 1 tbsp. oil to coat bottom of shallow baking dish. Roast loin 30 minutes per pound at 350 degrees to internal temperature of 145 degrees.

Allow the meat to rest for 10 minutes or more when it comes out of the oven. Divide the loin into two larger portions and one smaller portion, as the pork is merely a flavoring for the pork fried rice.

For the Purée

Each serving of pork is 4 oz. protein with one half cup sauce for the purée.

To create the purée, use either the barbecue sauce or the mushroom gravy. (See below).

Cut the pork into one inch pieces and place in the bowl of a mini food processor or the small pitcher of a blender with double rows of blades, such as the Ninja.

Pulse a few times to break up the protein and incorporate with the sauce.

Purée until smooth. Add mashed sweet potato or applesauce, ¼ cup to the purée, if you would like a sweet component to balance the dish.

The sides are a green vegetable such as spinach, mixed greens or garlic green beans. See Veggie Recipes.

If you make corn in the electric pressure cooker, one half cup of softened corn may be mixed with 2 tbsp. sour cream and 2 tbsp. milk to make creamed corn. The corn and the sour cream and milk are puréed in mini food processor or the blender. See recipe.

The loin of pork is an example of the Essential Purée technique of batch cooking. Once you make the loin of pork, you can make several meals out of it.

This is a good idea for stocking the freezer with good meals, labelled, with a USE BY date, listed on a white board. Saves time and labor.

The recipe calls for 2 lbs of pork loin.

Cut ½ lb. for making the pork fried rice and the wonton soup. Use ¼ lb. for each recipe. You can freeze the cooked pork until you are ready to have a Chinese takeout night at home. You know what's in the dish. Less fat and less salt.

After reserving the pork for the Chinese dishes, you will have one and ½ lbs. left. This amounts to six servings.

Make half with the mushroom gravy and half with the barbecue sauce.

You will have three servings of each. Freeze in individual portions.

Sides with the pork and mushroom gravy would be mashed sweet potato and greens.

Sides with the BBQ loin of pork would be creamed corn or mac and cheese and garlic green beans.

Cook once, eat three times. Variety is wonderful.

See Chinese dishes for purée instructions.

Barbecued Loin of Pork

PER SERVING

Calories	252
Fat	7 g.
Saturated Fat	2 g.
Sodium	565 mg.
Sugar	16 g.
Carbohydrate	20 g.
Fiber	0 g.
Protein	24 g.

Prep Time: 5 minutes
Cook Time: 10 minutes
Level: Easy
Serves 4

Ingredients

- 1 lb. cooked pork loin, cut into one inch cubes for purée

The Sauce

The sauce for purée is barbecue – store bought or homemade.

Barbecue is one of the most recognizable flavors for purée. I use a prepared barbecue sauce and two slices of pork per serving. At the moment, my favorite prepared sauce is Stubbs Honey Pecan. This creates a great purée.

A quickie homemade barbecue sauce: Always good in a pinch and made from pantry items:

In a saucepan, one cup of ketchup, one half cup molasses, two tablespoons of Dijon mustard, a shot of soy sauce, a tablespoon of honey and the secret ingredient of two tablespoons of hoisin sauce. This last ingredient may sometimes be found in the ethnic foods section of the supermarket, or in an Asian market. It is made from plums and imparts a rich deep flavor to the sauce. It is also slightly sweet and contains sugar. Diabetics, take note. I like the balance of the honey and the mustard, but if you wish, you can use brown sugar for the sweetener. All of this is according to taste and may be adjusted. If you prefer a mustard-based barbecue sauce, eliminate the ketchup and use only a tablespoon.

Stir all ingredients together over a low heat.

For the Purée

Combine the pound of pork with 1 cup of the BBQ sauce and pulse. Add an additional sauce as needed for smoothness of texture, usually ½ additional sauce but up to two cups. The object is to break down the protein in the sauce.

Variation

If pulled pork sandwiches are a big favorite in your house, you can buy a small pork butt or shoulder, cover with two bottles of store-bought mild barbecue sauce and cook low and slow in a slow cooker for six to eight hours, until the meat can be easily shredded.

For the Purée

Take 3/4 cup of pulled pork 2 tbsp. of milk BBQ sauce and 2 tbsp. of water.

Pulse until the pork is broken down. Purée until smooth. Add 2 tbsp. of broth, if needed for the purée.

As a side: In a NutriBullet nutrition extractor, extract a cup of store bought cole slaw from the deli section of your supermarket. Add a tablespoon of sour cream or low fat sour cream to dilute vinegar component and render the dish creamy.

After a 30 second extraction, the cole slaw will be rendered into a smooth liquid.

To make sure there are no particles of cabbage or carrot, please run it through a mesh sieve with a silicone spatula.

The liquid will contain the extracted veggies.

Thicken to correct level of the NDD diet with an instant thickener.

Serve pork in one dish and cole slaw in another, separately.

Loin of Pork with Mushroom Gravy

Prep Time: 15 minutes
Cook Time: 5 minutes
Level: Easy
Serves ?

Calories	297
Fat	27 g.
Saturated Fat	4 g.
Sodium	3 mg.
Sugar	1 g.
Carbohydrate	11 g.
Fiber	1 g.
Protein	3 g.

This is a classic brown gravy with vegetables added. This gravy beats anything you can buy in the supermarket. It has low sodium and no chemicals and preservatives. You can control the ratio of vegetables to liquid. It is a great way to get extra vegetables into the diet.

Gravy is important. This is how you get flavor into the dish and get the correct texture in the protein.

Ingredients
- 1 lb. cooked loin of pork

The Sauce
- 1 cup mushrooms
- 4 tablespoons oil, can be extra virgin olive oil or canola oil
- 1 teaspoon fresh thyme, minced
- 2 tablespoons Wondraflour, from the supermarket
- 1 cup simmering water or lower sodium broth
- Pan juices from the roast pork.

Directions
Mince a handful of baby portobellos or any combination of mushrooms you like. A cup of mushrooms will do for a cup of liquid.

Cut off the nubby end of the stem and wipe the mushroom clean with a damp paper towel. Slice the mushrooms into medium slices. You may remove the stems and use them in the warmed liquid, creating a more intense flavor, a mushroom stock.

The baby portobellos, Baby Bellas, have more flavor than the white button mushrooms.

Sauté in 1 tablespoon olive oil. Add 1 tsp. minced fresh thyme from the herb garden. Alternatively, a pinch of dried thyme will work. Mushrooms will soak up the oil. Add the second teaspoon if pan gets dry. If pan continues to get dry, use a tablespoon of broth of any kind at a time. This will only impart flavor to the mushrooms. The choice for Essential Purée is always lower sodium broth, when using store bought broth. Not every cook has time to make the broth at home, although it is well worth while to put this on your cook's schedule.

Remove mushrooms from pan with any juices and reserve in a bowl.

In the sauté pan, add two tablespoons oil and two tablespoons Wondraflour and brown the flour. I use Wondraflour because it is light and contains rye flour and gives a good quality gravy. Also, it has less tendency to lump.

When roux has browned, about a minute and a half, slowly add one cup simmering water. Whisking is a good idea. Stir or whisk as you go, careful to keep the gravy free of lumps.

Add mushrooms back to gravy. Cook for about six minutes, to allow gravy to thicken and cook out the raw flour taste. This finishes the cooking of the mushrooms.

Yield: Single recipe yields two one-half cup servings of gravy.

The meal: The protein serving is 4 oz. of pork and ½ cup of gravy. The sides are mashed sweet potato and braised greens or any other green vegetable. (See Veggie Recipes)

Note: This beats anything you can buy packaged and off the shelf or in the freezer. It is fresher, it is of higher quality and it is cheaper. It also tastes fabulous and not like an overly processed mush. My mother ate with great enthusiasm and did not lose weight.

Hint: Double the recipe is you want to have extra gravy on hand in the freezer.

Tip: This freezes really well in one cup servings, which is enough for a purée of one serving.

Tip: If more liquid is needed for purée, use a little water or stock. Taste as you go. You do not want to lose the flavor of this dish by adding too much water. If necessary, mix the sweet potatoes in the purée. The object is to get the smooth, creamy consistency.

Onion and Pepper Smother Gravy

Yield: Two Servings of gravy

PER SERVING	
Calories	198
Fat	14 g.
Saturated Fat	2 g.
Sodium	367 mg.
Sugar	3 g.
Carbohydrate	15 g.
Fiber	1 g.
Protein	4 g.

A classic flavor profile and a time-honored favorite of Italian street food as served in the fantastic onion sausage and pepper sandwiches at the San Gennaro Festival in New York City. Adapted for home use.

Ingredients

- ½ yellow onion, sliced into thin half moons
- ½ red or green bell pepper or a combination of any of the bell peppers, sliced into thin half moons
- 2 tablespoons olive oil
- 2 tablespoons Wondraflour from the supermarket
- 1 teaspoon lower sodium soy sauce
- ¼ teaspoon of white pepper (better texture for swallow)
- 1 cup of lower sodium chicken stock or vegetable stock at the simmer, meaning bubbles around the edges of the saucepan.

Directions

Pan sauté the onions and peppers in the olive oil. Remove from pan.

Add two tablespoons oil and flour and brown the flour about a minute and a half to take away the raw flour taste.

Slowly add the simmering broth, stirring as you go. Add the soy sauce and the seasonings.

Sauce will thicken in about a minute or two. Add the onions and mushrooms back in.

For the Purée

The meal: 4 oz. pork, one half cup gravy. And one half cup braised greens or braised cabbage, see Veggie Recipes. Serve ½ cup of applesauce on the side with the pork dish.

I always add an extra vegetable whenever possible. It is excellent in terms of nutrition and deepens the flavor.

Hint: Double the recipe if you want to store gravy in individual portions of one half cup in the freezer. The rule of thumb is a half cup of purée liquid to a 4 oz. serving of protein, adding extra water or stock if needed. The trick is to get the protein into a smooth consistency. The drippings from the roasting make a big difference.

 Tip: When you have frozen homemade gravy on hand for purée, you can use the sauce with any other protein such as a chicken breast or a small steak (4 oz. portion). You can even use it to purée a burger.

On the Go

This is a great meal to take "on the go" for travel or for family events such as celebrations or cookouts. Take a frozen meal.

Purée the meal in advance, add instant thickener to stabilize, and freeze it in a glass container.

For the trip: Simply take along a small cooler and place the frozen meal in the bag.

In a restaurant or airport, simply ask if the restaurant will thaw the meal in the microwave at 50% power. Stir it and serve.

If the meal is not puréed. Think about bringing along a Nutribullet in a transport bag. In the portable bag, you can bring along eating utensils and envelopes of instant thickeners and thickened water or even thickeners for various types of drinks. You can also bring along a container of pudding for dessert

Pork Fried Rice: Chinese Takeout at Home

Prep Time: 15 minutes
Cook Time: 15 minutes
Level: Easy
Serves 4

The meal: Pork Fried Rice and Stir Fry with a bowl of Won Ton Soup.

This is meant to be your Chinese takeout meal in a healthy form. This has far less sodium and oil than typical takeout.

Ingredients

- 2 cups cooked rice (See Whole Grains Recipes)
- 1 carrot sliced into half moons, or a handful of baby carrots, sliced on the bias to increase the surface area
- 3 scallions, sliced thinly
- 1 clove garlic, sliced thinly
- ½ cup frozen peas
- 4 oz. slices loin of pork, cut into small dice (about four slices of ¼ inch)
- Lower sodium soy sauce (to taste)

Directions

Sauté sliced scallions until translucent, about a minute.

Add carrots and sauté, about two minutes, adding a little water to steam the carrots into softness

Add garlic at the end and sauté for one minute, to prevent burning.

Stir in cubed pork.

Add cooked rice, and stir fry with vegetables and pork, giving rice a chance to pick up flavor and be coated with oil.

Add about a quarter cup of water and about 2 tbsp. lower sodium soy sauce, for flavor and color. One may use chicken stock or vegetable stock instead of water.

Again stir fry the rice and lower the heat and allow the rice to steam into softness and rehydrate.

For the Purée

Warm the cooked rice through with additional broth until it is hydrated and soft.

Add a cup of the warmed and hydrated fried rice to the bowl of a mini food processor or to the small pitcher of a double-bladed blender.

Pulse six to eight times to break down the elements of the dish.

Purée until smooth. Add warm broth, or water, as needed to get your needed consistency.

The rice turns into almost a porridge. This form of rice porridge is called congee and it is used throughout Asia to feed the very young and the elderly. It has nutritional content and it has fiber. With the soft-cooked protein and the soft cooked vegetables, it has flavor as well as nutrition. The rice forms a base for the purée of the protein. It might not require any instant thickener.

The meal: Use one cup of Wonton Soup (See Soup Recipes) and 1 cup of fried rice with one cup of stir fry (See Recipe).

Technique Note: Stir fry is a method of cooking that uses high heat and moves the food around in the oil for a sear and then finishes by braising with a liquid. You can do it in a sauté pan or a regular wok, but I use an electric wok because I love it.

Ingredient Note: The classic prep for fried rice is to add bean sprouts and a scrambled egg at the very end. I eliminate the sprouts because of their stringy texture. Sprouts may be difficult to swallow. Also, because I store the food in the fridge and in the freezer, I eliminate the egg for reasons of food safety. If one wants to add extra protein at time of service, scramble an egg separately and stir into fried rice before purée.

 Tip: I use brown basmati rice because it is easier for my mother to digest. It is light and aromatic in the cooking. I use a rice cooker or an electric pressure cooker to soften the rice. (See Whole Grains for cooking directions). I do not, under any circumstances, use white rice or instant rice of any kind. The nutritional value is diminished by the processing.

Batch Cooking

I make two cups of rice at a time in the pressure cooker. I freeze it in half cup portions. I date it and add a USE BY date for thirty days. I have a handy component for a meal to go along with a protein in gravy. Add it to your white board.

When I use the rice, I warm it through in broth or gravy to thoroughly soften the rice.

Then I add the half cup of rice with the broth or the gravy to the bowl of a mini food processor or the small pitcher of a blender.

I pulse a few times to get the purée going.

I purée until the rice is smooth. The rice may be served separately because it has flavor.

It may also be added to the dish that includes a serving of protein with a serving of sauce or gravy.

Variations

As anyone who has ever eaten in a Chinese restaurant knows, you can vary the fried rice by varying the protein. Pork, chicken, shrimp, scallops or any other leftover protein will do. Protein amounts are the same. For vegetarians, use firm tofu.

Shrimp Stir Fry

Prep Time: 10 minutes
Cook Time: 10 minutes
Level: Easy
Serves 2

PER SERVING

Calories	370
Fat	18 g.
Saturated Fat	3 g.
Sodium	691 mg.
Sugar	3 g.
Carbohydrate	7 g.
Fiber	1 g.
Protein	45 g.

Ingredients

- 1 lb. of shrimp, either fresh or frozen. If tail on, remove tails after cooking
- 1 clove garlic, minced
- 1 inch slice ginger, peeled and minced
- 2 scallions, sliced thinly
- 1 medium zucchini, cut into quarter moon slices for fast stir fry
- 3 tbsp. water for steaming zucchini
- 3 tbsp. Soy Vay Veri Veri Teriyaki Sauce or Soy Vay Hoisin Garlic Asian Glaze (see Tip on next page)
- 2 tbsp. peanut oil

Directions

If using cooked frozen shrimp, thaw in a bowl of ice water, drain and pat dry before adding to dish. If using fresh shrimp, wash, pat dry and de-vein, using a knife along the back of the shrimp. I cook with tail on for flavor and remove tail for purée.

Heat 1 tbsp. peanut oil in a wok or a large skillet. If using cooked shrimp, simply stir the shrimp in oil to warm it and remove to a plate. If using uncooked shrimp, stir, heat 1 tbsp. oil in wok or large skillet. Add the aromatics, the garlic, ginger and scallion. Stir fry for two minutes. (I usually remove the ginger after the sauté, as I do not purée it with the dish. If patient does not like ginger, please eliminate it.)

Add the shrimp and stir fry until the shrimp turn pink. A few minutes. Remove from pan and reserve, keeping warm.

Add the zucchini, stir fry for two minutes, add the water, cover, and steam the zucchini until soft, about four minutes. Add more water if need be to complete cooking.

When zucchini is soft, add the shrimp back in, add the sauce, whichever you prefer and stir until well combined.

For the Purée

Add one cup of the stir fry to the bowl of a mini food processor or to the small pitcher of a blender.

Pulse several times to break up the veggies and the shrimp.

Purée until the dish is smooth. Wipe down the sides of the pitcher or the sides of the bowl, if necessary, with a rubber spatula so that all of the dish goes through the blades.

Because of the sauce and the zucchini, this purées very nicely. Add a little water if you need it to get a smooth purée of the protein.

Safety Note: I serve the second portion within three days when stored in the fridge. I freeze this dish for a maximum of two weeks.

Variation

Can be made with bay scallops. I keep a bag of frozen ones in my freezer for alternate source of protein.

Tip: I use the Soy Vay brand because it is readily available in supermarkets and is made without stabilizers, gums or artificial ingredients.

Barbecue Pork in the Slow Cooker

PER SERVING

Calories	277
Fat	9 g.
Saturated Fat	3 g.
Sodium	753mg
Sugar	14g
Carbohydrate	15 g.
Fiber	0 g.
Protein	32 g.

Prep Time: 5 minutes
Cook Time: 6 hours
Level: Easy
Serves 6

Ingredients

- 2 lbs. pork shoulder or butt
- 1 bottle Stubb's original barbecue sauce
- 1 and ½ cups water
- 1 tablespoon hoisin sauce
- 1 tablespoon molasses
- 1 tablespoon Dijon mustard
- 1 tablespoon ketchup
- 1 teaspoon soy sauce

Directions

Place pork and all the sauce ingredients in a slow cooker. Cover and cook on low for six hours.

The pork should pull apart for pulled pork sandwiches. The reason I use Stubb's is that it is a mustard based barbecue sauce and is not loaded with a high sugar content. It has plenty of good flavor and a clean heat. For a change, I use Stubb's honey pecan.

Check with your healthcare provider to make sure the individual is cleared for the sauce.

For the Purée

Place 3/4 to 1 cup of pulled pork plus ½ cup of sauce in the bowl of a mini food processor.

Pulse to break up. Purée. Use instant thickener if needed to bind the dish.

Grilled Lamb Chops with Mashed Potatoes

Prep Time: 10 minutes
Cook Time: 16 minutes for medium rare
Level: Easy
Serves 2

Calories	212
Fat	12 g.
Saturated Fat	3 g.
Sodium	72 mg.
Sugar	0 g.
Carbohydrate	1 g.
Fiber	0 g.
Protein	23 g.

Ingredients

- Four lamb chops
- 2 cloves garlic
- 1 tablespoon olive oil
- 1 sprig rosemary, chopped
- Salt and white pepper

Directions

Preheat grill. I use High to get the best sear on the meat.

1 recipe mashed potatoes, or leftover mashed potatoes. (See Veggies).

Make a marinade of the grated garlic, the rosemary and the olive oil, salt and white pepper.

On an indoor grill, or under the broil, cook the lamb chops to desired doneness. I make mine medium rare. It is best to cook lower and slower to keep meat tender and flavorful.

Variation

Use a thicker chop, boneless, but cook it tender. Using 2 tbsp. vegetable oil, sear 2 chops on either side for two minutes until golden. Use a medium high heat. Do not char.

Remove from pan and reserve on a plate.

Slice one yellow onion in half, then slice one half in quarter inch slices. Core and seed one green pepper. Slice in quarter inch slices.

Stir fry the onions and peppers in a tablespoon of vegetable oil over medium high heat.

Return pork chops to the pan. Add a quarter cup water or broth and two tablespoons lower sodium soy sauce.

Lower heat to simmer and cover the pan.

If you have a freezer portion of the smother gravy, defrost it and use it for the braising liquid. If you have the extra frozen gravy from the pot roast, defrost in the microwave and use that for the braising liquid.

Allow the chops to braise for fifteen minutes, adding gravy, water or broth if needed. Check for doneness with a thermometer. 145 degrees.

The dish is done when the pork is cooked to your desired doneness. Vegetables will be soft.

For the Purée

Allow the chops and the veggies to cool.

Take one of the chops and chop it up and place it in the bowl of a mini food processor or the small pitcher of a blender. Add ¼ cup of the braising liquid.

Pulse six times until the pork breaks up.

Add one half cup of the braising liquid and vegetables.

Pulse until combined with the pork.

Purée until smooth, adjusting liquid. This is your main dish.

Thoroughly mix a ½ cup serving of mashed potatoes with ¼ cup of smooth gravy. Serve as a side dish.

You could also use a ½ cup serving of pressure-cooked rice combined with a ¼ cup broth or gravy and puréed until smooth in the bowl of a mini food processor or the small pitcher of a blender.

Veal Marsala

Prep Time: 15 minutes
Cook Time: 12 minutes
Level: Intermediate
Serves 2

PER SERVING

Calories	167
Fat	4 g.
Saturated Fat	1 g.
Sodium	348 mg.
Sugar	2 g.
Carbohydrate	6 g.
Fiber	1 g.
Protein	27 g.

Ingredients

- 8 oz. veal cutlets
- 8 oz. mushrooms, your choice, sliced
- 2 tbsp. olive oil for sauté
- ¼ cup Marsala wine
- ¼ cup chicken broth (lower sodium)
- 1 tbsp. chopped parsley

Directions

Trim any silver skin off cutlets or they will be sinewy. If veal cutlets are not of even thickness, place them between two sheets of plastic wrap and gently pound them with a small kitchen mallet.

Season with salt and white pepper. Heat 2 tablespoons of olive oil.. Brown two minutes per side in the pan. Remove from pan.

Add oil and sauté the mushrooms. Add the chicken broth and the Marsala wine, and add veal back to pan.

Cook for five minutes, turning once. Add parsley for the last minute.

The sauce will be thin. If serving to the rest of a family, thicken with two teaspoons of flour in a tablespoon of water, to make a slurry. After removing veal and mushrooms from pan, add the slurry, let the gravy come to a simmer and cook for four minutes to take away the raw taste of the flour.

For the Purée

Allow the dish to cool. Cut up 4 oz. of the veal. Add it to the bowl of a mini food processor or the small pitcher of a blender. Add 2 tablespoons of the gravy.

Pulse 10 times to break up the veal, adding more liquid if necessary.

When the veal is smoothly puréed, add ½ cup of mashed potatoes combined with ¼ cup of Marsala gravy.

Tip: When in need of a quick recipe of mashed potatoes, try Edward & Sons Organic Mashed Potatoes. Ready in five minutes. Superior to supermarket brands. No chemicals or preservatives. Clean eating.

Chicken Marsala

Prep Time: 15 minutes
Cook Time: 12 minutes
Level: Intermediate
Serves 2

Calories	174
Fat	4 g.
Saturated Fat	1 g.
Sodium	338 mg.
Sugar	2 g.
Carbohydrate	6 g.
Fiber	1 g.
Protein	28 g.

Ingredients

- 8 oz. skinless, boneless chicken breasts
- 8 oz. mushrooms, your choice, sliced
- 2 tbsp. olive oil for sauté
- ¼ cup Marsala wine
- ¼ cup chicken broth
- 1 tbsp. chopped parsley

Directions

Butterfly the breasts by cutting them in half horizontally, so they will not be too thick. If the chicken breasts are not of even thickness, place them between two sheets of plastic wrap and gently pound them with a small kitchen mallet.

Season with salt and white pepper. Heat 2 tablespoons of olive oil. Brown two minutes per side in the pan. Remove from pan.

Add oil and sauté the mushrooms. Add the chicken broth and the Marsala wine, and add chicken back to pan. Cook for five minutes, turning once. Add parsley for the last minute. The sauce will be thin. If serving to the rest of a family, thicken with two teaspoons of flour in a tablespoon of water, to make a slurry. After removing the chicken and mushrooms from pan, add the slurry, let the gravy come to a simmer and cook for four minutes to take away the raw taste of the flour.

This is delicious puréed with one half cup mashed potatoes and ¼ cup of sauce.

For the Purée

In the bowl of a mini food processor or a blender with double blades, place 4 to 6 ounces of chicken, broken up.

Add ¼ cup of sauce

Pulse five times to break down the chicken.

Purée until smooth.

Add to bowl. Use a tablespoon of instant thickener to bind the dish.

The side dish is one half cup of mashed potatoes combined with ¼ cup of gravy. See recipe.

You can thicken the purée with several tablespoons of mashed potato.

 Tip: When in need of a quick recipe of mashed potatoes, try Edward & Sons Organic Mashed Potatoes. Ready in five minutes. Superior to supermarket brands. No chemicals or preservatives. Clean eating.

Cod Cake

(Baked Fish with Homemade Mashed Potatoes)

PER SERVING

Calories	121
Fat	1 g.
Saturated Fat	0 g.
Sodium	63 mg.
Sugar	0 g.
Carbohydrate	7 g.
Fiber	1 g.
Protein	21 g.

Prep Time: 5 minutes
Cook Time: 10 to 12 minutes
Level: Easy
Serves 2

I include tilapia, halibut, snapper, mahi mahi, and grouper. I use fresh frozen wild salmon for my Salmon in Puff Pastry. The best is fresh fish.

Ingredients

- 8 oz. fresh cod
- 2 tbsp. olive oil
- Salt and white pepper
- 1 lemon

Directions

Preheat oven to 350 degrees.

Season the cod and lay two thin slices of lemon on top. Bake in a 350 degree oven watching it, until fish is firm to the touch and flaky. Remove from oven.

For the Purée

The trick to puréeing fish is to have a medium that purées well. Homemade mashed potatoes have the perfect texture. The way to keep the flavor at the maximum is to have the right proportion of fish to mashed potato. A half cup of mashed potato to a five ounce serving of fish is about right. The result is creaminess. See the recipe for Mashed Potato.

When cool, remove lemon slices. Break up the fish in the bowl of a mini food processor. Add several tbsp. of the pan juice. Pulse until smooth. Add a half cup of Mashed Potatoes and purée for 10 seconds until combined. Do not over purée or you will get gummy potatoes.

Serve with a half cup of puréed garlic green beans on the side.

Tip: Another way to prepare the cod is to lay the fish on a piece of foil, season with salt and white pepper, add a dash of olive oil and two slices of lemon. Seal the foil packet. Steam for 10 minutes in a steamer, until fish is cooked through.

Tip: I know the recipe says Homemade Mashed Potatoes, but sometimes you need a shortcut. Sometimes you have to get a meal on the table. Don't feel guilty. This is the best way to do it. When in need of a quick recipe of mashed potatoes, try Edward & Sons Organic Mashed Potatoes. Ready in five minutes. Superior to supermarket brands. No chemicals or preservatives. Clean eating.

Salmon in Puff Pastry

Prep Time: 25 minutes
Cook Time: 30 minutes
Level: Medium
Serves 4

PER SERVING

Calories	483
Fat	15 g.
Saturated Fat	3 g.
Sodium	141 mg.
Sugar	0 g.
Carbohydrate	32 g.
Fiber	2 g.
Protein	28 g.

This is basically a fish pie. I like it because it has a protein, a carb and a green all in one dish. My mother and I used to go to a local restaurant that served salmon cakes in lemon sauce and it was a favorite of hers. I created this dish because she liked the salmon cakes and the flavor profile was familiar to her.

I know how to make Alfredo from scratch, but I am often time-challenged. I use a store bought alfredo and doctor it with lemon juice and a shot of Tabasco. The sauce serves as the medium for the purée and carries the flavor. Salmon of course contains healthy omega-3s, and I use fresh spinach. If there is a time constraint, I use frozen spinach. I use store bought puff pastry.

This dish freezes beautifully. I wrap each individual portion in plastic wrap and then aluminum foil and then enclose it in an individual plastic container. My freezer is like a pantry. Each individual serving of any dish is labeled with instructions for serving and a USE BY date.

This recipe is for four servings. The sauce makes an excellent purée. Two servings go in the fridge and two in the freezer.

Ingredients

- Store bought puff pastry sheets from freezer section of market. Thawed in refrigerator. One sheet.
- Two filets of salmon, 8 oz. each
- Two cups cooked rice (See recipe in whole grains)
- 1 shallot, thinly sliced
- 1 clove garlic, thinly sliced
- 1 bunch spinach, washed and drained. Alternatively, a half bag of frozen spinach.

Directions

Preheat oven to 375 degrees

In a sauté pan, cook the thinly sliced shallot until soft but not caramelized. Sauté the thinly sliced garlic for a minute. Add spinach to the pan.

Marinate salmon fillets in two tablespoons lower sodium soy sauce, two tablespoons lemon juice, salt and white pepper to taste, in a plastic sip bag, in fridge, for one hour.

Wilt spinach in the pan in a tablespoon of safflower or grapeseed or extra virgin olive oil. Lightly season with salt and white pepper and a shot of lower sodium soy sauce.

Remove from pan. Drain extra liquid and reserve. Does not have to be drained dry as liquid aids in purée.

The Rice

I make rice in the electric pressure cooker or in the rice cooker for the softest texture. I freeze individual servings in glass covered storage dishes. If the rice needs hydrating when defrosted, place a tablespoon of oil in a pan, add the rice and add several tablespoons of broth or plain water. Stir. Allow the rice to absorb the water or broth and soften. Then use it.

To Compose the Fish Pie

Arrange the dish. Line a sheet pan with parchment paper or a silicon liner. Lay out one sheet of puff pastry. Arrange the rice in a square down the center, leaving enough pastry to fold up and enclose. Take cooled, drained spinach mixture and place on top of rice. Arrange salmon fillets end to end on top of spinach.

Enclose the three layers in the puff pastry and squeeze the edges shut. Leave a hole open at the center for escaping steam. Brush the puff pastry with egg wash, meaning an egg beaten with a tablespoon of water.

Bake in oven until pastry is golden brown, approximately 30 minutes. Check after 20 minutes. If puff pastry is browning, cover with aluminum foil to protect it. Salmon is done when knife goes into firm flesh and is warm to the touch when it comes out.

Remove, let cool before slicing.

For the Sauce

These days it is possible to buy good store bought Alfredo in a variety of flavors. Pick one you like. Add two tablespoons of lemon juice to brighten it up and thin it out.

For the Purée

Slice the loaf into four servings, each approximately four ounces of salmon. Break up the loaf into the bowl of a mini food processor or the small pitcher of a blender with double blades.

Add ½ cup of sauce.

Pulse to break up the components of the dish.

Purée until the dish is smooth.

You have the protein, the carb and a green vegetable in one delicious dish.

Crab Cakes

Prep Time: 45 minutes
(15 minutes hands on, chilled in fridge for half hour)
Cook Time: 10 minutes
Level: Medium
Yield: 6 servings of two small crab cakes

Calories	226
Fat	17 g.
Saturated Fat	2 g.
Sodium	692 mg.
Sugar	1 g.
Carbohydrate	8 g.
Fiber	1 g.
Protein	10 g.

Ingredients

- ½ lb. jumbo lump crab meat
- ½ cup bread crumbs (store bought)
- 1 small diced red onion
- ½ small diced red pepper
- 2 stalks of tender heart of celery, finely diced
- 1 one half inch slices of ginger, grated into the onion as it sautés
- 1 teaspoon lemon or lime juice
- 1 shot Worcestershire sauce (or to taste)
- 2 eggs, beaten lightly
- ½ cup good mayonnaise
- 1 teaspoon Dijon mustard or horseradish Dijon, if you like spicy
- Salt and White Pepper to taste
- 1 tsp. Old Bay seasoning
- 1 tsp. finely chopped chives
- 1 tsp. finely chopped flat leaf parsley
- 1 tbsp. olive oil for vegetable sauté
- ¼ cup fine ground corn meal for dusting the crab cake

Directions

In a tablespoon of vegetable oil, sauté the onion and ginger for two minutes, to flavor the oil.

Add the red pepper and celery and continue sautéing until all the vegetables are soft. About 10 minutes.

Add the lemon juice (or lime), Tabasco and Worcestershire sauce with the Old Bay seasoning. Add the chopped herbs.

Using low heat, cook spices for 1 minute with the veggies. This gives a depth of flavor and removes any raw taste. Remove from pan to a bowl and allow to cool.

In a separate and non-reactive bowl, preferably glass, porcelain or stainless steel: Beat the eggs lightly until lemony yellow. Add the mayonnaise, mustard, and bread crumbs to the mixture, add the cooled veggies with seasonings and finally fold in the crab, being careful not to break it up. This should hold together and not be too loose to form cakes. You want the mixture loose to hydrate the bread crumbs. Chill the mixture for half an hour to allow it to firm up.

Remove from the refrigerator. Form patties using an ice cream scoop to measure and form patties with your hands. Do not pack the crab mixture tightly.

Line a baking sheet with parchment paper or a silicone liner. Bake cakes in a 375 degree over for 10 minutes. You can dust them lightly with finely ground corn meal before baking.

I like to make smaller cakes, 2 inches in diameter, to make sure they heat through.

For the Purée

Take two crab cakes and break up in the bowl of a mini food processor or the small pitcher of a blender. Add three tablespoons of warm water or warm broth.

Pulse four or five times to break up the crab cake. Check to make sure there is no graininess.

Purée to smooth texture.

Remove from bowl. If desired, mix thoroughly with a half cup of mashed potatoes from the recipe in the Veggie section.

Tip: When in need of a quick recipe of mashed potatoes, try Edward & Sons Organic Mashed Potatoes. Ready in five minutes. Superior to supermarket brands. No chemicals or preservatives. Clean eating.

Black Bean Crab Cakes

PER SERVING

Calories	349
Fat	25 g.
Saturated Fat	4 g.
Sodium	627 mg.
Sugar	2 g.
Carbohydrate	16 g.
Fiber	1 g.
Protein	15 g.

Serves 4

This is the Asian flavor profile. In one of my favorite Chinese restaurants in San Francisco, the house specialty is crab cakes in black bean sauce. This is a rendition of that recipe in a crab cake. Flavor of this dish is smoky.

Ingredients

- ½ lb. jumbo lump crab meat
- ½ cup plain bread crumbs
- 3 thinly sliced scallions
- 1 stalk tender heart of celery, finely diced
- 1 one-inch slices of ginger, grated
- 1 clove garlic, grated
- 1 teaspoon black bean and garlic sauce
- 1 tablespoon mirin (Japanese product found in Asian section of grocery)
- 1 tablespoon fresh lemon juice (or rice vinegar)
- ½ cup good mayonnaise
- 2 lightly beaten eggs

Directions

Sauté the aromatics and veggies in a tablespoon of peanut oil or canola oil. This would be the ginger, scallions, garlic, red pepper and celery and let them cool. Add the black bean sauce, mirin and lemon juice. Gently stir and heat through over low heat. Remove from heat and allow to cool.

Mix all remaining ingredients thoroughly but gently in a non-reactive bowl, such as porcelain or stainless or glass. Chill for thirty minutes in refrigerator.

Use an ice cream scoop to measure out crab cake. Form crab cakes with a loose pack. Place on parchment lined sheet pan. Heat oven to 375 degrees. Cook crab cakes for 10 minutes. To keep the cakes warm, they can be held in a 250 degree oven..

Purée using ¼ cup seafood stock or vegetable stock. Add a small amount at a time and pulse slowly.

Pulse food processor or blender slowly so as to be gentle with the crab.

For the Purée

Place two crab cakes in the bowl of a mini food processor or the small pitcher of a flat-bottomed blender. Add ¼ cup seafood stock or vegetable stock. Add a small amount at a time and pulse to combine into a smooth texture.

The Sides

For an Asian style side dish, stir fry half an onion, thinly sliced, add one cup of thinly sliced Napa cabbage. Stir fry for two minutes, then add ¼ cup of stock and simmer until tender, about five minutes. This sauteed cabbage side may be placed in the small cup of a nutrient extractor such as a NutriBullet or a NutriNinja and liquefied. Use ½ tablespoon of instant thickener to thicken. Add in half tablespoon increments until the cabbage purée is the correct thickness for your level of the NDD.

◎ **Tip:** For a good lower sodium soy sauce, I buy a brand called San-J, which is a Tamari sauce, gluten free, and reduced sodium, with excellent flavor. This is available in the Asian section of many supermarkets and also in the natural foods store. For black bean sauce, I use Lee Kum Kee variety (available in grocery stores in the Asian section or in specialty markets or online.)

A Taste of South Beach:

Stone Crab and Baked Potato Cakes

PER SERVING

Calories	162
Fat	8 g.
Saturated Fat	1 g.
Sodium	652 mg.
Sugar	1 g.
Carbohydrate	11 g.
Fiber	1 g.
Protein	12 g.

I grew up in Miami Beach and have been eating stone crabs at Joe's Stone Crab, the famous restaurant at the end of the beach, all of my life. In season for part of the year and expensive, the Florida stone crab has a unique flavor. I think it is the best crab in the world. At Joe's, one of the classic sides for "stonies" is baked potato. Joe's serves a mustard sauce that is the perfect complement to the crab. I have given the classic recipe, with a salute to the great watering hole.

Ingredients

- One pound of stone crab claw meat
- 2 tablespoons of good mayo mixed with
- 1 tablespoon of Dijon mustard
- 1 tablespoon of sour cream.
- 1 and ½ cups of the flesh of two medium sized baked potatoes.

For the Purée

In the bowl of a mini food processor or the small pitcher of a blender, add mayo, mustard and sour cream. Pulse two or three times to combine.

Break the flesh of the potatoes into the bowl. Blend the potato with the sauce by pulsing five times. Add the stone crab and blend the potato with the sauce. Give the stone crab the least amount of buzz in the food processor to obtain the desired texture.

This will give you a great purée.

A side of creamed spinach is traditional with stoned crabs.

Lasagna

Prep Time: 30 minutes
Cook Time: 50 minutes
Level: Intermediate
Serves 6

Calories	484
Fat	14 g.
Saturated Fat	8 g.
Sodium	329 mg.
Sugar	10 g.
Carbohydrate	61 g
Fiber	4 g.
Protein	27 g.

Ingredients

- 1 quart tomato sauce, either homemade or store bought
- 1 package Barilla no-boil lasagna noodles, or homemade noodles if you like

Filling

- 3 cups part skim ricotta cheese
- ½ cup grated parmigiano reggiano
- 2 extra large eggs, lightly beaten
- Salt and white pepper to taste
- 2 tbsp. Gourmet Garden parsley paste

I make one layer, as one layer of noodles is sufficient for purée. More layers create more noodles and the consistency of the purée becomes too thick.

Directions

Preheat oven to 350 degrees.

In a bowl, mix the ricotta and the parmigiano. Add the eggs and check the consistency of the filling, using a few tablespoons of milk to get a smooth and creamy consistency. This is, in essence, a cheesy custard, and will set up well.

Put a cup of sauce in the bottom of your lasagna pan. I use a 9 x 13 baking pan or for smaller lasagnas, a 9 x 9. Either way.

If you are adding ground meat or sausage, this is the time to add it to your sauce.

Create the bottom layer of noodles, allowing the noodles to overlap one another slightly to create a solid base.

I add a little extra sauce on top of the bottom layer of noodles, not to soak the noodle, but to make sure it cooks properly.

Layer in the filling. Add a small amount of sauce and vegetables to the top of the filling, again for the purpose of making sure the noodles cook properly.

Layer the top layer of noodles. Add a cup of sauce, smoothed over the surface and add your vegetables here, mushrooms, or spinach and artichoke, or sautéed zucchini.

Sprinkle with parmesan cheese and bake in oven for 50 minutes, until bubbly. Remove from oven and let cool.

Note: I eliminate the traditional mozzarella cheese in my lasagna because of potential for swallowing difficulties. The various ingredients may be layered in the sauce for variety, nutrition and depth of flavor.

For the Purée

This purées beautifully. It also freezes beautifully. I put small containers of sauce in the freezer for the purpose of purée, in case it is needed. This is to eliminate the necessity of thawing a quart container of sauce for a mere several tablespoons of puréeing liquid.

Please note: The process of puréeing adds air to the ricotta cheese mixture and increases the volume of the dish. One serving looks like more than one serving.

In puréeing for the meal, I cut out the square for one serving about six inches square. So the dish does not look huge, I reserve some of the square and serve the amount that one serving normally occupies in the bowl. Otherwise, the patient is overwhelmed and takes a long time eating. If my mom is still hungry, I bring more food. Or I give her a snack.

Note: Aside from the convenience of using no-boil lasagna noodles, I also use them because they are thinner. The purée is better with the thinner noodle. The proportion of carbohydrate to protein and vegetable is better for nutritional balance. I tried it both ways, and found that the no-boil noodle was less starchy and gummy in the purée. Just make sure you have enough sauce below and above to cook it well.

Variations on Lasagna

As You Like It

The lasagna basic recipe uses only cheese for protein. You can add either vegetables or sautéed and browned meat for extra oomph. Let your palate be your guide.

- 1 cup sautéed mushrooms, seasoned with fresh thyme can be added to the sauce.
- One large zucchini, sliced lengthwise, into one quarter inch slices. If you are good with a knife, use a chef's knife. If not, use a mandolin or a counter top slicer for even slices. This will allow the zucchini to cook at the same rate. Zucchini gives off a little water, so sauté well and pat dry if necessary before adding to recipe. Sauté zucchini with a little sliced garlic, salt and white pepper can go on top of the filling.
- 1 can artichoke hearts, quartered, washed, drained and dried or 1 package frozen artichoke hearts, quartered, can also go into the sauce.
- 1 lb. spinach, wilted in a sauté pan and pressed dry, can be added to the sauce
- Spinach and artichokes can be added to the sauce together.

Meat: ½ lb. Italian sausages, hot or sweet, with meat extracted from the skin and browned in a pan

Or ½ lb. of ground beef or turkey or chicken, browned in a pan can be added into the sauce.

For the Purée

Adding any of these ingredients to the sauce will not affect the purée. The meat or veggies cook tender because of the oven time.

Using the mini food processor or the small pitcher of a double bladed blender, place the serving in the appliance. Pulse several times to break down the dish. Then purée until smooth.

Mom's Meat Loaf Updated

Prep Time: 20 minutes
Cook Time: 50 minutes
Level: Easy
Serves 4

PER SERVING

Calories	199
Fat	10 g.
Saturated Fat	3 g.
Sodium	186 mg.
Sugar	1 g.
Carbohydrate	4 g.
Fiber	1 g.
Protein	22 g.

Meat Loaf is the ultimate American comfort food. A diner classic. Served with a side of Mom's mashed potatoes and Diane's garlic green beans.

Ingredients

- 1 lb. package ground turkey
- ½ onion, diced finely
- 1 clove garlic (grated)
- 2 tbsp. Gourmet Garden parsley paste
- 2 tbsp. parmesan cheese
- 1 egg
- ¼ cup bread crumbs
- ½ tsp. salt and ¼ teaspoon white pepper
- A sprinkle of olive oil for moisture, as turkey is low in fat
- A shot of Worcestershire sauce
- A shot of lower sodium soy sauce
- A shot of extra virgin olive oil for richness

Directions

The base: sauté the onion, garlic and carrot in a tablespoon of olive oil. Add a tablespoon of water to steam until veggies are tender. Allow to cool.

In a bowl, add the ground turkey and the fresh parsley, parmesan cheese, bread crumb and the beaten egg. Wet the bread crumbs with water and squeeze excess water out.

Add the cooled veggies.

Combine turkey, veggies, egg, seasonings and breading, very lightly mixing with hands. Form loaf and put on a baking sheet or in a shallow baking dish that has been coated with a little oil. Form loaf lightly and do not pack.

Top with half a cup of ketchup. This prevents the meat loaf from drying out. This is optional.

Cook at 375 degrees for fifty minutes or until juices run clear. Allow to stand for 10 minutes.

Then slice and serve with mashed potatoes and garlic green beans or slice for sandwiches.

For the Purée

I use two slices per purée with one half cup of mashed potatoes and a couple of tablespoons of homemade gravy.

Purée with homemade gravy. Or with gravy and mashed potatoes. In a pinch, you can substitute store bought gravy, but often these are high in sodium, so read your labels. The brown gravy is standard American diner fare, but one can use tomato sauce for gravy as well.

Yes, you can purée a sandwich. Use only one slice bread, add the favorite condiment, whether mayonnaise or ketchup and the slice of meat loaf. Purée a side of cole slaw.

 Tip: For those on gluten free diets, use half a cup of old-fashioned oats as binder.

Variation

Substitute ground chicken or ground sirloin or a mixture of beef and pork for protein.

The Freeze

This dish freezes well. I use to put two slices, with a half cup of mashed potatoes and a half cup of gravy in the container for the freezer. In a glass storage dish, place two slices of meat loaf with half a cup of mashed potatoes and half a cup of gravy. The food is pre-measured, ready to thaw and purée.

Steak Chili

Calories	273
Fat	12 g.
Saturated Fat	3 g.
Sodium	283 mg
Sugar	6 g.
Carbohydrate	23 g.
Fiber	6 g.
Protein	21 g.

Prep Time: 15 minutes
Cook Time: 1 hour
Level: Easy
Serves 6

Ingredients

- 1 lb. steak, ribeye or sirloin, cut into one-inch cubes
- 1 medium yellow onion, diced
- 2 cloves garlic, sliced thinly
- 2 tbsp. tomato paste whisked with either red wine or water
- 1½ tsp. chili powder
- ½ tsp. cumin
- 2 dashes Tabasco (optional)
- ¼ tsp. cayenne powder (optional)
- Salt and white pepper to taste
- 2 tbsp. olive oil
- 1 28 oz. can crushed tomatoes with purée
- 1 8 oz. can tomato sauce
- 1 15 oz. can lower sodium kidney beans, rinsed and drained (optional)

Directions

At room temperature, trim excess fat and rub the steak with salt and white pepper. Cut the steak into half inch cubes. Brown the steak in olive oil and remove from pan, keeping any remaining juices.

The base: sauté the onions until translucent, add the garlic and saute for one minute, add the chili powder, cayenne, Tabasco, cumin to brown the spices and then add the thinned out tomato paste. At this point, add a dash of Worcestershire sauce if you like it.

Add the meat to the base. Add the crushed tomatoes and the tomato sauce and the beans. Stir well and add water to desired looseness if the chili is too tight. Simmer for an hour.

Note: The heat in this chili is very mild. Please get clearance from your healthcare provider

For the Purée

After chili has cooled to a warm temperature, add 1 cup to the bowl of a mini food processor or the small pitcher of a blender. Add toppings of choice, including finely grated cheddar cheese that will melt with the heat of the chili, even in a warm state. Also, another favorite topping, tablespoon of sour cream.

A tablespoon of finely minced red onion is also permissible if your machine will purée it.

To be sure of rendering raw onion into a purée, use a high speed blender (Vitamix or one of the newer less expensive clones) or a nutrition extractor (NutriBullet or NutriNinja.)

Purée until smooth.

Bind the chili with instant thickener, 1 pump or 1 scoop. Purée for 10 seconds to thoroughly combine.

Tip: This is the classic chili with an upscale twist. For traditional chili texture, substitute ground beef or ground turkey. Just season and brown the ground meat and proceed with the recipe.

Tip: I usually make corn bread to go along with the chili and purée a small slice in with the chili. Store bought corn bread is fine. With the rest of the corn bread, one can make desserts, using it as the base for strawberry shortcake or peach crumble (see Desserts). Freezes beautifully when wrapped first in plastic wrap and then in foil then in covered plastic container.

Blond Chili

PER SERVING

Calories	183
Fat	11 g.
Saturated Fat	2 g.
Sodium	65 mg.
Sugar	4 g.
Carbohydrate	8 g.
Fiber	2 g.
Protein	14 g.

Prep Time: 10 minutes
Cook Time: 1 hour
Level: Easy
Serves 6

Ingredients

- 1½ pounds chicken breast, cubed into inch-cubes. Use a combination of light and dark meat if desired. (breast may be ground in the Ninja with pulsing)
- 1 medium yellow onion, diced
- 2 cloves garlic, sliced thinly
- 2 tbsp. tomato paste whisked with either red wine or water
- 1½ tsp. chili powder
- ½ tsp. cumin
- 2 dashes Tabasco (optional)
- ¼ tsp. cayenne powdered (optional)
- Salt and white pepper to taste
- 2 tbsp. olive oil
- 1 28 oz. can crushed tomatoes with purée
- 1 8 oz. can tomato sauce
- 1 15 oz. can cannellini or white kidney beans, rinsed and drained (optional)

Directions

Follow directions for steak chili. This blond chili is lighter, with a tomato base.

If you really want to make this a blond chili, use chicken broth and thicken it, or take a can of cream of chicken soup (I get mine from the organic section of the supermarket) and use that as your base. You come up with a blond sauce. Add a tablespoon of green chillies to for the heat. This you get in the Latin food section of your supermarket. If you use chili powder, it will make the chili red. Ditto the Tabasco, unless you use the green Tabasco. This is mild, but get approval of healthcare provider.

Veggie Chili

Prep Time: 15 minutes
Cook Time: 1 hour
Level: Easy
Serves 6

Calories	165
Fat	4 g.
Saturated Fat	1 g.
Sodium	214 mg.
Sugar	6 g.
Carbohydrate	27 g.
Fiber	6 g.
Protein	10 g.

Ingredients

- 6 oz. Tempeh, cut into half inch cubes
- 1 red onion finely diced
- 1 clove garlic
- ½ jalapeno pepper, no seeds or stem or ribs, fine dice
- 1 sautéed red pepper
- 2 cups sautéed kabocha squash
- 3 large Portobello mushroom sautéed
- 2 leeks, white parts only, cleaned and sautéed
- 1 15 oz. can diced tomatoes with garlic and basil
- 1 small can tomato sauce
- ½ can tomato paste, thinned with water
- 1 15 oz. can black beans.
- 1 tsp. chili powder (optional)
- Dash Tabasco sauce (optional)
- 2 dashes Worcestershire sauce
- 2 tbsp. red wine, if alcohol is permitted

Directions

In the bottom of a 5 or 8 quart soup pot or in the bottom of a slow cooker that has a skillet function, sauté tempeh in 2 tbsp. oil plus two tbsp. lower sodium soy sauce. In other words, for a meatless recipe, use tempeh just as you would ground meat. Remove and hold to one side.

Sauté all the vegetables, then add the diced tomatoes, tomato sauce and tomato paste, as well as the rest of the seasonings.

There are no rules as to the number of vegetables you can add. The object is a medley of flavors and textures. If you like, you can add a half cup of thinly sliced carrots or parsnips to the veggie sauté. Whatever is your favorite.

Cook in slow cooker for an hour. The longer the cooking, the more developed the flavors. The squash will impart body to this dish and give it some backbone.

For the Purée

Allow to cool. Add one cup veggie chili to the bowl of a mini food processor or the pitcher of a blender.

Top with ¼ cup shredded cheddar cheese and 1 tablespoon sour cream, and a sprinkle of slivered scallions. Here is where you add extra protein. If you like it, add firm tofu in one inch squares. The chili will heat the tofu.

Purée until smooth. Stabilize the purée with one pump or one scoop of instant thickener. Purée 10 seconds to combine.

Prep note: To my taste, Kabocha is the most delicious of all the varieties of squash in the entire squash world. The flavor is superb. It is a Japanese variety. During the autumn that I lived in a Japanese house in Tokyo, I kept a whole shelf of them so I would have them for making miso soup. Kabocha has a unique texture and makes a terrific purée. I like it best with skin removed. It is worth the extra step to prepare it separately.

Cut squash into quarters, remove seeds and webbing, and cut each quarter into one inch squares, sauté and then add a cup of broth or water to simmer until tender. Ten minutes. Let cool. Remove the green skin. Add to the chili.

Flavor Note: The Portobello mushrooms serve as the biggest texture and are reminiscent of meat. If you long for a meaty weight to the chili, add more portobellos.

Note: Tempeh is a protein source made from organic soybeans with millet, brown rice and barley. It has a nice flavor and texture and is a traditional protein source for vegetarians from the cuisine of Indonesia. I have used the brand manufactured by LightLife which is available in whole foods stores. Can keep in the refrigerator or freezer according to package directions.

Stuffed Cabbage

Prep Time: 15 minutes
Cook Time: 1 hour
Level: Medium
Serves 4

Calories	412
Fat	10 g.
Saturated Fat	3 g.
Sodium	145 mg.
Sugar	15 g.
Carbohydrate	51 g.
Fiber	6 g.
Protein	27 g.

This may seem like an old-fashioned dish, but think of it as a warm wrap baked with a sauce. The classic green to use for the wrap is cabbage, but there is no reason that the wrapper could not be kale or chard. The world of sauces then opens up and so does the world of flavor profiles. I also like it with kasha as the grain.

Ingredients

- 8 leaves of green cabbage or Napa cabbage, cored, washed and dried
- 1 15 oz. can of tomato sauce

Filling

- 2½ cups cooked rice
- 1 lb. ground sirloin or pork, or chicken or turkey
- ½ medium yellow onion, diced
- 1 clove garlic, minced
- 2 tbsp. fresh parsley, cut finely

Directions

Preheat oven to 350 degrees.

Parboil cabbage leaves in a few quarts of water for three minutes or steam them in a steamer for three minutes. Allow to cool.

In a sauté pan, cook onions until translucent, about two minutes, add the clove of garlic. If you wanted to add julienned carrots, this would be the moment.

Add the rice and the parsley and stir in veggies, combining well. I like to add in about 2 tbsp. water to help reconstitute the rice, if it has been frozen. This re-hydrates each kernel of rice and gives it the consistency of a risotto, without the aggravation. A shot of lower sodium soy given the rice a good flavor.

The Cabbage Rolls

On a clean cutting board, center a cabbage leaf. Add about three or four tablespoons of the filling in the center in the shape of a log. This is just like rolling a little log of sushi or a spring roll.

Bring the edge of the cabbage leaf over the filling and tuck the end down. Roll in the two sides, and complete the rolling of the stuffed cabbage log. If you wish, you may anchor the top in place with a toothpick.

Line up the completed cabbage logs in a baking dish, I use a 9 x 9 square for two rows of four. Cover with tomato sauce. Add a bay leaf to the sauce for flavor, if you like.

Cover with foil and bake in 350 degree oven for one hour. You have protein and carb and one veggie. Easy to purée with sauce.

This can be made vegetarian by substituting finely diced firm tofu for ground beef.

For the Purée

When the dish cools, break up one or two cabbage rolls and place in the bowl of a mini food processor or a blender.

Add one half cup of sauce.

Pulse five times to break up the components of the dish.

Purée until smooth. Check to make sure that the cabbage has puréed smoothly.

If necessary, pass through a mesh sieve using a silicone spatula.

To bind the purée, add one scoop or one pump of instant thickener. Combine thoroughly.

Diane's Stuffed Portobello Mushrooms

Prep Time: 15 minutes
Cook Time: 12 minutes
Level: Intermediate
Serves 4

Ingredients

- 4 big Portobello mushrooms, wiped with a damp cloth
- Olive oil, salt and white pepper for seasoning

Filling

- 1½ cups wilted spinach, kale or chard (deveined)
- 2 shallots or a quarter cup yellow onion sliced thinly
- ½ cup mascarpone cheese
- ¼ cup parmigiano reggiano
- Sixteen medium shrimp, cooked, deveined, tail off

Directions

Paint the bottom of the mushroom with a brush dipped in olive oil. Put salt and white pepper in the olive oil and perhaps a splash of lower sodium soy sauce.

Line the mushrooms on a baking sheet, cap side down.

For the filling

Sauté the onion or shallot in a tablespoon of olive oil in a pan until translucent, about a minute or two.

Wilt the spinach, chard or kale. If using chard or kale, remove the tougher stems with a knife. Chiffonade the greens before cooking. This means rolling them up like a cigar and slicing into ribbons.

After cooking, press out excess liquid in a strainer with the bottom of a spoon. Reserve the liquid in case it is needed for the purée.

Add drained chopped greens to the ricotta and parmesan and mix with the beaten egg, salt and white pepper. (As an alternative to ricotta, use ¼ cup of mascarpone).

Slide into 400 degree oven for twelve minutes. At this point, the mushroom will be tender.

Add the cooked shrimp on top, four large ones to a mushroom, more if the shrimp are smaller.

For the Purée

Allow the mushrooms to cool.

Slice the stuffed mushroom in four pieces and place in the bowl of a mini food processor or a blender. If there are mushroom juices in the pan, add these to the blender. Add liquid from greens if needed to get desired consistency.

To bind the purée, add one scoop or one pump of instant thickener. Combine thoroughly.

Tip: I like to take the gills out of the portobellos when I stuff them. Use the tip of a spoon and scrape gently. Wipe off the mushrooms with a damp paper towel to clean them. This is for better texture and color, and gives more room for the filling.

Tip: Scallops may be added to these mushrooms. Marinate and sauté for a couple of minutes to a side, so that scallop is done. Should be firm to the touch. Do not overcook or scallop will be tough. This is a way of adding extra protein to the dish. Lump crab meat may also be added. Since it is cooked, it does not have to be cooked again. Because of the inclusion of shellfish, this is a festive dish and I often serve it at the holidays in the days before the service of a major holiday meal. It makes a nice lunch on New Year's Day.

Holiday Ham with Pineapple Honey Mustard Glaze

PER SERVING

Calories	467
Fat	18 g.
Saturated Fat	4 g.
Sodium	243 mg.
Sugar	51 g.
Carbohydrate	55 g.
Fiber	2 g.
Protein	25 g.

Prep Time: 15 minutes
Cook Time: According to weight of ham
Level: Intermediate
Yield: 1 serving as follows:

The Protein

For this dish, in our small household, I bought my ham from the deli counter in the market rather than baking an entire ham.

For a holiday meal with a whole family, buy and prepare a ham according to directions. Most holiday hams come in 10 pound sizes. So if you only need a few servings, I have been advised by my butcher that the best holiday ham for a small serving of five pounds is a bone-in smoked ham. This is pre-cooked. I heat it according to directions for the weight of the ham. I plan to serve two portions and freeze two portions, so I use a pound of ham for four servings.

The Glaze

I prepare my own glaze. There are a number of store-bought glazes, especially at the holidays. You can use them, but I find they are often too heavy on the spices for the patient with swallowing difficulties. They contain preservatives and chemicals and the homemade version does not.

- 4 oz. fresh pineapple, cored, or one 8 oz. canned pineapple with natural juices.
- 4 tbsp. honey
- 1 tbsp. Dijon mustard
- Sprinkle of cinnamon and a tiny dash of cloves

Purée the pineapple in its juices and add the honey and mustard and spices. Cook for five minutes to bring the glaze together. Paint the ham with half of this when it is warmed on a sheet pan in a low oven of 200 degrees. Reserve the rest of the glaze to add flavor to for purée. As it is high in sugar, use a tablespoon for flavor.

For the Purée

For the purée: two ham slices cut into one inch squares go into the Ninja.

This is for a four ounce serving of protein. Add one tablespoon of the glaze and a half cup of the mashed sweet potato recipe. Buzz until smooth.

To bind the purée, add one scoop or one pump of instant thickener. Combine thoroughly.

Serving the Meal

The main dish is ham and sweet potato with a veggie on the side.

The Main Course:

- Two slices ham, 4 oz., cut into half inch cubes
- One half cup mashed sweet potato with orange recipe
- 1 tablespoon glaze

This gives a smooth creamy consistency to the purée and has a nice contrast in flavor between the sweet and the salty. A tablespoon of the glaze is good to start with then if you need more liquid, use a tablespoon of water at a time.

The Sides:

Make a recipe of braised greens for the side dish and purée with its liquid.

Another great side dish is a recipe of the garlic green beans..

Tip: The puréed dish of ham and sweet potatoes with glaze freezes beautifully, so you can do two portions at once and have one on hand in the freezer.

Roast Turkey Breast with Lemon and Herbs

Prep Time: 20 minutes
Cook Time: 2 hours
Level: Easy
Serves 8

PER SERVING

Calories	212
Fat	14 g.
Saturated Fat	3 g.
Sodium	105 mg.
Sugar	0 g.
Carbohydrate	0 g.
Fiber	0 g.
Protein	20 g.

A turkey breast is more manageable than a whole bird. If you like dark meat, use the same herbs, but buy a package of legs.

Ingredients

- 1 turkey breast, 6 lbs.
- Zest of half a lemon
- 3 tbsp. olive oil
- 2 tbsp. finely chopped rosemary, fresh
- 2 tbsp. finely chopped flat leaf parsley, chopped
- 3 tablespoons finely chopped sage, fresh, chopped
- 2 tbsp. thyme leaves, fresh, chopped

Directions

In the bowl of a mini food processor, combine olive oil, lemon zest and herbs into a paste. Loosen the skin at the opening of the large cavity. Apply the herb paste under the skin. On top of the skin, apply either butter or olive oil, massaging it in, and liberally salt and white pepper.

Place breast on rack in roasting pan. Add 1 cup chicken or turkey stock and ½ cup white wine to the roasting pan. This will give you pan juices for later.

Place roasting pan in center of 325 degree oven and cook for two hours. Thermometer inserted into thickest part of breast should read 160 degrees.

Halfway through the cooking, if the skin is browning too much, cover loosely with aluminum foil.

Remove breast from rack and let rest on cutting board for fifteen minutes. Slice against the grain.

Pan juices can be placed in gravy boat and served with a ladle to the family, and used for purée for the person with swallowing difficulties.

A serving is a four ounce portion of turkey puréed with ½ cup of mashed potatoes and ¼ to ½ cup of turkey gravy. If you like cranberry sauce, get your favorite and add a tablespoon to the purée, for the complete holiday flavor profile.

For the Freezer:

Take two slices of the roast turkey, about 4 ounces, and freeze with a half to a whole cup of Homemade Turkey Gravy. Then your entrée is ready to go.

Homemade Turkey Gravy

This can be made from pan juices and turkey stock. The method is the same as for the brown gravy. Using two tablespoons of good oil and two tablespoons of flour, brown the flower in the oil. Add a cup of simmering stock a little at a time, whisking to prevent lumps. Then add a second batch of the herbs as listed in ingredients, or just the parsley and thyme, or some poultry seasoning from the spice rack and stir for a minute in the simmering gravy to cook them.

When the gravy cools, run it through a mesh sieve to remove any pieces of herbs and any lumps.

For the Purée

Allow the turkey to cool while you make the homemade turkey gravy from the recipe on this page. Remove a cup of the gravy from the pan and place it in a measuring cup and allow it to cool.

When turkey is cool, slice it down. One serving of protein is four ounces. Two servings is eight ounces. Cut up the turkey meat and add it to the bowl of a mini food processor or the small pitcher of a blender, preferably one with double blades.

Pulse 10 times to break up the turkey. Add gravy, a tablespoon at a time to aid in this process if necessary.

Add the rest of the ½ cup of gravy and purée to combine. To bind the purée, add one scoop or one pump of instant thickener. Combine thoroughly. This is the first part of the dish.

In a second serving dish, add a serving of puréed cranberry sauce. Make sure the cranberry sauce is puréed to smooth texture, in a nutrition extractor if necessary.

For a half cup of cranberry sauce, thicken with a pump or a scoop of instant thickener. Use a half teaspoon for a tablespoon of cranberry sauce.

Once the sauce is puréed, it may be frozen for adding to dishes.

The third part of the dish:

If you have made the Mashed Potatoes with a potato ricer and they are completely smooth, then take a half cup portion of mashed potato and sir in one or two tablespoons of gravy.

As long as all three components of the holiday meal are the same thickness, there should be no problem for the swallow. The vegetables are puréed separately and served in separate dishes. This adds to the color of the meal.

Veggies

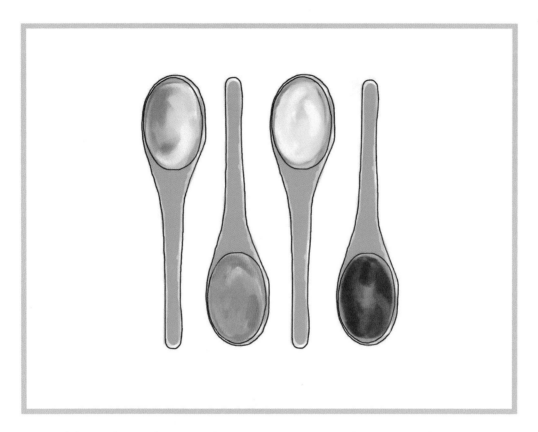

Vegetable cookery shows real mastery. I use a wide variety of vegetables of all colors, to get in all the phytochemicals. I think they are fabulous enough to carry an entire meal and they taste wonderful when mixed together or in combination with whole grains.

Slow-Baked Sweet Potatoes with Orange

PER SERVING

Calories	86
Fat	3 g.
Saturated Fat	0 g.
Sodium	30 mg.
Sugar	1 g.
Carbohydrate	14 g.
Fiber	2 g.
Protein	1 g.

Prep Time: 10 minutes
Cook Time: 90 minutes
Level: Easy
Serves 4

The sweet potato is loaded with nutrients and is a favorite in our house. We like it flavored with orange and cinnamon, to add a little tartness as a balance to the sweet. I bake three or four good sized potatoes at a time, for the four servings. This is easy.

Ingredients

- 4 medium sweet potatoes, approximately the same size (1 and a half lbs.)
- 2 tbsp. olive or vegetable oil
- 2 tbsp. orange marmalade (preferably lower sugar)
- 2 tbsp. orange juice
- Shake of cinnamon

Directions

Preheat oven to 300 degrees

Wash and dry potatoes and cut off sharp ends or blemishes.

Puncture each potato three times with knife to allow steam to escape.

Put oil in a shallow bowl and brush outside of potato with oil.

Cover with aluminum foil. Line up on baking sheet, leaving distance between for air to circulate.

Bake 90 minutes, until potatoes are soft. Remove from oven and allow to cool enough to handle.

Open foil and remove skins, placing potato in bowl.

For the Purée

Run the sweet potatoes one cup at a time through a potato ricer to remove any fibers remaining in the potato.

Return to the mixing bowl.

To the marmalade, add two tablespoons of warm water and run through a mesh sieve to remove any zest of the orange.

Add the marmalade and the orange juice to the riced sweet potato. Add the cinnamon. Combine thoroughly using a fork.

Tangerine juice may be substituted for orange juice.

For additional sweetener:

Sometimes sweet potatoes need sweetening. A tablespoon of honey dissolved in a tablespoon of warm water may be added. Stevia to taste may be added. Brown sugar to taste may be added.

The sweet potato purée should now be a smooth creamy pudding consistency.

The batch of sweet potato should be divided into individual servings in glass storage containers, dated, and put in the freezer. The USE BY date is for one month.

8 servings. 2 servings go in fridge, each dated for one week.

 Tip: This is an excellent medium for purée for all sorts of savory dishes, as it gives any protein a creamy consistency.

Diane's Homemade Mashed Potatoes

Calories	87
Fat	4 g.
Saturated Fat	3 g.
Sodium	55 mg.
Sugar	1 g.
Carbohydrate	10 g.
Fiber	1 g.
Protein	3 g.

Prep Time: 15 minutes
Cook Time: 20 minutes
Level: Easy
Yield: 4 one-half cup servings

This recipe can be doubled.

Who would think that making mashed potatoes involves cooking technique. I give you a choice to save time and labor.

There are two ways to make potatoes for this recipe. One is the old-fashioned way of boiling them in a pot of salted water. This takes twenty minutes and you have to peel the potatoes. The second way is to use an electric pressure cooker. This takes seven minutes and renders the potatoes very soft. A four-quart pressure cooker is plenty big enough and is an excellent tool for the dysphagia kitchen.

Technique is also important for puréeing the potatoes. Use a potato ricer or a food mill. If you use a mini food processor to blend the potatoes with a protein, process the protein first, so it is puréed. Add the potato at the very end, perhaps with a few tablespoons of broth or gravy, for creaminess, flavor and texture. Watch the potatoes as the sharp blades of the food processor will cut the molecules in such a way that you have created a dish that has the texture of library glue. This is not good for the swallow. You will have to throw it away. Be warned! Technique is everything when it comes to the humble but delicious comfort food of mashed potato.

Ingredients

- 1 pound potatoes, gold or red
- Water to cover potatoes
- Salt

Directions

Peel your potatoes and cut them into equally sized pieces. Cover with cold salted water, bring to the boil and cook for twenty minutes until fork tender.

Drain and return to pot to make sure potatoes are dried out.

When potatoes cool, put them through a potato ricer. This is the easiest and the fastest way to get smooth potatoes in a purée.

For the Mash

Once potatoes have been through the potato ricer, add:

- 2 pats of butter or margarine (2 tbsp.)
- ½ cup of warm milk
- 1 scant tablespoon of good mayonnaise or Lemonaise mayonnaise substitute
- Salt and white pepper to taste

Stir all ingredients together until well combined and fluffy.

Tip: One way to get very tender mashed potatoes is to cook two pounds of potatoes with a cup of water for 7 minutes.

If you use regular sized potatoes, cut them into quarters. I like baby Yukon Gold potatoes because they do not have to be cut up. The Yukon Gold potato has a creamy texture when cooked.

When the potatoes cool, using a kitchen towel, wipe them and remove the skins. Discard the skins. Put the potatoes through a potato ricer and then follow the directions for the mash. This is easy and convenient.

It is best not to put potatoes through a food processor. They may get gummy. This is not desirable for the swallow.

Tip: The mashed potatoes freeze better when mixed with a gravy or a protein and a gravy. When I make such dishes as the lamb chops or the crab cakes, I purée the protein in the bowl of a mini food processor or a high speed blender. I then combine thoroughly with the mashed potato. Protein and potato may then be frozen.

Creamed Corn

Prep Time: 10 minutes
Cook Time: 5 minutes
Level: Easy
Serves 4

PER SERVING

Calories	134
Fat	6 g.
Saturated Fat	2 g.
Sodium	20 mg.
Sugar	3 g.
Carbohydrate	18 g.
Fiber	2 g.
Protein	3 g.

Corn makes an excellent side carbohydrate in place of rice, potatoes, quinoa, couscous or pasta. In summer, I use fresh corn on the cob. In winter, I buy organic frozen corn in the whole foods store and prepare it in the electric pressure cooker. Corn is a whole grain, the grain of the Americas, as it is the premier food discovery of the New World. I mean no disrespect to the tomato.

Ingredients

- 4 ears of fresh corn on the cob
- 1 cup water
- Salt, 1 tsp.
  Optional: ¼ cup of milk (My father always swore by adding a little milk to the boil. I believe the lactic acid softens the corn.)

Directions

Equipment: An electric pressure cooker renders the corn tender for the purée.

Place corn kernels and one cup water and half a cup of milk if desired into the electric pressure cooker. Cook for six minutes. With a sharp knife, remove kernels from cob.

In a frying pan, add a pat of butter or non trans-fat margarine or a tablespoon of good vegetable oil. Swirl kernels around. Add ¼ cup lower fat sour cream and three tablespoons of milk to thin. Add white pepper to taste.

For the Purée

Place a cup of the corn and cream sauce in the small cup of a nutrition extractor. Buzz for 10 seconds, until completely smooth.

Add a pump or scoop of instant thickener to stabilize the dish.

Note: Freezing the cobs allows one to use them later for fish or shellfish stock.

Grilled Summer Vegetables

Calories	39
Fat	0 g.
Saturated Fat	0 g.
Sodium	5 mg.
Sugar	4 g.
Carbohydrate	9 g.
Fiber	2 g.
Protein	2 g.

Prep Time: 20 minutes
Cook Time: 30 minutes
Level: Easy
Serves 4

This purées beautifully and is a great side dish.

Ingredients

- 1 lb. mushrooms, baby bellas, wiped with a damp cloth and de-stemmed
- 2 medium zucchini, cut in half vertically and sliced into rectangles about ¼ inch thick, about a pound
- 2 onions or a bunch of scallions, sliced into ¼ inch rounds
- 2 red bell peppers, cored and seeded with ribs removed, sliced into ½ inch wedges

Directions

Heat grill to indoor 375 degrees or High setting.

Placed sliced vegetables in a bowl and coat with a swirl of olive oil. Add salt and white pepper. Place vegetables in rows on the grill and cook, approximately 3 to four minutes to the side in case of the mushrooms, and two to three minutes for the rest, to desired doneness.

This makes four good servings of vegetables. For the purée, add water and perhaps a touch of fresh lemon juice. Vegetables will be tender and will need small amount of water to purée. Taste is excellent.

Goes beautifully with a piece of grilled fish and mashed potato or a turkey burger and extracted and thickened cole slaw. This is a classic Italian starter.

Tip: I use an indoor electric grill. I live in Florida and it is too hot to grill outside in the summer. The indoor grill has the benefit of easy clean-up. Also, I do not have to deal with charcoal or propane in order to get a meal on the table. A number of good ones are on the market.

Roasted Winter Vegetables

PER SERVING

Calories	173
Fat	1 g.
Saturated Fat	0 g.
Sodium	143 mg.
Sugar	15 g.
Carbohydrate	4 1g.
Fiber	9 g.
Protein	4 g.

Prep Time: 30 minutes
Cook Time: 1 hour
Level: Easy
Serves 4

Ingredients

- 1 butternut squash, peeled and cubed into two-inch cubes (about 1½ pounds)
- 1 sweet potato, peeled and cut into two inch cubes
- 2 leeks, cut into two inch sections, white parts only
- 3 cloves garlic, peeled
- 3 carrots, cut into two-inch sections
- 1 parsnip, cut into two-inch pieces
- 3 small white turnips, sliced into quart-inch slices
- 3 small beets, sliced into quarter-inch slices

Directions

Preheat oven to 400 degrees.

Prepping the vegetables takes the longest with this dish, but it is well worth it.

By using an entire butternut squash, you get the makings of a butternut squash soup as a bonus side dish.

Prepare two baking sheets. I usually line mine with aluminum foil. The first contains mixed vegetables. The second contains the other half of the butternut squash.

Lay the mixed vegetables out on the first sheet and the second half of the butternut squash and any extra veggies on the second. If you do not have leeks, use a yellow onion or shallots, which roast beautifully. I reserve the green part of the leeks for creating homemade soup stock.

Put sheets into oven and roast. After thirty minutes, I sprinkle the veggies with a little water in order to keep them moist. If they appear to be drying from the heat, cover them with a little foil after adding the water.

For the Purée

Place sheet pan of vegetables on a trivet and allow to cool.

Remove the flesh of the butternut squash from the skin and discard the skin or compost it.

Remove the flesh of the sweet potato from the skin and do the same.

Choose some of each vegetable and break up and place in the bowl of a mini food processor or of a blender. (Sometimes I make a purée of butternut squash by itself or with leek.)

Add a little broth or water to the bowl or the pitcher.

Pulse the vegetables a few times to break up. Purée until smooth. Add more liquid as needed for the purée.

If you wish to bind the vegetable dish or if you need to firm it up for the swallow, add instant thickener at this point and purée until combined.

The butternut squash on the second rack can be puréed to soup consistency. Use water for intensity of veggie flavor. As my mother was a pulmonary patient, I tried to cut back on dairy, but the dish can be puréed with milk or even cream for those with no problem with dairy. The object here is to get two or even three dishes from one session of cooking.

I often use this as the base for one of my quiches, which is made with the butternut squash purée and sautéed mushrooms, with a little goat cheese (chevre) or a little Swiss or Gruyère, whatever you happen to have on hand. Quiche purées beautifully.

Tip: I use a small Chinese cleaver to cut the butternut squash in half vertically, as it requires muscle power. Insert the tip of the cleaver at the top of the squash and lean firmly as you lower the cleaver down the neck and into the body of the vegetable. Simply leveraging your weight ought to do it. If the peel resists the application of a knife down the outside of the vegetable, then remove the skin after roasting when it is soft.

Diane's Butternut Squash Quiche

Prep Time: 20 minutes
Cook Time: 50 minutes
Level: Medium
Serves 8

PER SERVING

Calories	221
Fat	13 g.
Saturated Fat	5 g.
Sodium	155 mg.
Sugar	1 g.
Carbohydrate	19 g.
Fiber	1 g.
Protein	6 g.

Ingredients

- 2 cups puréed butternut squash, cooked
- ¼ cup milk (could substitute water for depth of veggie flavor)
- 4 eggs, lightly beaten
- ½ cup yellow onion, thinly sliced
- ½ cup of sautéed mushrooms, cooked in a tablespoon of olive oil and a splash of lower sodium soy sauce
- 1 prepared pie crust or make your own
- 4 oz. of softened chevre cheese or ¼ cup grated Gruyère or Swiss cheese
- 1 tablespoon fresh thyme

Directions

Preheat oven to 375 degrees.

Saute the onions in a tablespoon of olive oil until they are lightly golden and translucent, about 3 minutes. When cool,place in the bowl of a mini food processor. Sauté the sliced mushrooms in a tablespoon of olive oil and add a dash of lower sodium soy sauce halfway through cooking. Allow to cool.

Place the mushrooms in the bowl of the mini food processor with the onions. Pulse a few times to break up vegetables. Then purée to a smooth consistency, adding warm water a tablespoon at a time if necessary

Prepare a quiche pan with a crust. I like to prick the crust and bake for 10 minutes at 375 before I add the vegetable custard. Let cool.

Purée the butternut squash with milk. Beat the eggs lightly. Add a splash of soy for flavor. Break up the goat cheese and add. It should be at room temperature. Add the thyme. I use my fingers to get the tiny thyme leaves off their tiny stems, and then bruise them with my fingers as I add them to the recipe. This allows them to release their essential oils.

Add the eggs and soy to the squash and mix gently. I mix the puréed onions and mushrooms into the quiche, add the cheese, and then fill the quiche pan. For added stability and ease of moving the quiche, put it on a sheet pan for transfer to oven.

Bake at 375 degrees for fifteen minutes until the quiche sets. Then lower heat to 350 degrees and cook for another 35 minutes until a knife goes in and comes out cleanly.

For the Purée

Slice the quiche. Remove the filling from the slice and place in a bowl. Since this was made with puréed veggies, and is a custard, this is good texture for the swallow.

If you wish to have crust, take the slice of crust and place it in the bowl of a mini food processor. Soften the crust with a tablespoon of warm broth. This takes less than a minute. Purée the crust until smooth. Add a half pump or a half scoop of instant thickener to bind the crust.

Place in a bowl next to the filling.

The bite is a third of a teaspoon of crust with two-thirds of a teaspoon of filling.

Tip: If I am time-challenged and do not have time to roast vegetables to make the quiche, I use a good butternut squash soup acquired from the whole foods store as my base for the quiche and leave out the ¼ cup of milk for purée.

Roasted Mushrooms

Prep Time: 10 minutes
Cook Time: 12 minutes
Level: Easy
Serves 4

Ingredients

- 1 lb. baby Portobello mushrooms, or any other type of mushroom
- 2 tbsp. olive oil
- Salt and white pepper to taste, ½ tsp. salt and ¼ tsp. white pepper, a shake of lower sodium soy sauce.

Directions

Preheat oven to 400 degrees.

Take a damp towel and swipe any dirt off your mushrooms.

Prepare a sheet tray by brushing a little olive oil on it.

In a bowl, mix the olive oil, salt and white pepper, and soy sauce if you are using it. Add the mushrooms and toss. Line up the mushrooms, cap side up, on the sheet tray.

Cook in the oven for twelve minutes, or until they reach desired tenderness.

For the Purée

When the mushrooms have cooled, break them up and add them one or two cups at a time to the bowl of a mini food processor or the small pitcher of a blender.

Pulse five to 10 times to break up the mushrooms.

Add broth one tablespoon at a time and purée until smooth.

If you wish to make a quickie mushroom gravy, add a tablespoon of sour cream, a tablespoon of broth, with a tablespoon of instant thickener.

Purée until combined, about 10 seconds. Adjust seasonings remembering to use white pepper. For an herbal flavor, use a half teaspoon of Gourmet Garden thyme paste, then purée

Tip: These are delicious puréed by themselves, using a little water if needed. They make a terrific accompaniment to any protein, but are especially good if you are puréeing a burger or a steak with mashed potatoes. Use them as a component if you are making a gravy or a pan sauce. Excellent frozen.

Tip: I am a mushroom fanatic and scour the farmer's markets for specialty mushrooms such as the delicious chanterelle or the ever popular and expensive morel mushroom. I like the Japanese varieties available in supermarkets such as the oyster mushroom or the enoki mushroom, or the Chinese straw mushroom which is better fresh than canned.

You can also use any specialty type of mushroom that happens to grow in your area, bearing in mind that cooking time might vary, as long as mushrooms reach desired tenderness for the purée. Just watch them, test them, and poke them. If mushrooms give up a liquid during cooking, by all means incorporate it into your purée for added flavor.

Roasted Asparagus

Prep Time: 10 minutes
Cook Time: 12 minutes
Level: Easy
Serves 4

PER SERVING

Calories	52
Fat	4 g.
Saturated Fat	1 g.
Sodium	2 mg.
Sugar	2 g.
Carbohydrate	4 g.
Fiber	2 g.
Protein	2 g.

Most people are familiar with steamed asparagus, but roasting them gives them intensity of flavor.

Ingredients

- 1 lb. asparagus (I prefer thick stalks to pencil asparagus for flavor. For the gourmet touch, use white asparagus in season.)
- 1 tbsp. olive oil
- Salt and white pepper to taste

Directions

Preheat oven to 400 degrees. Prepare a baking sheet by covering it with parchment paper.

Rinse asparagus and pat dry. Snap off tough ends of stalks. In a bowl, add asparagus, olive oil, salt and white pepper and toss with your hands.

Line up stalks on baking sheet. Pope into oven and roast for 12 minutes until tender.

For the Purée

The best tool for puréeing asparagus is the nutrition extractor such as a NutriBullet or a NutriNinja.

Break up the asparagus and place them in the small cup, or the bowl of a mini food processor or the small pitcher of a blender.

If you use a food processor or a blender, to make certain that all fibers are removed from puréed asparagus, run the purée through a mesh sieve with a silicone spatula.

Add a scoop or a pump of instant thickener to bind the purée.

Tip: I like to cook two batches of the recipe at once, so I have a delicious ingredient to add a little zing to my classic recipes. The idea is that it is better to cook once and have the ingredient for multiple uses. Roasted asparagus will bring a depth of flavor to any dish that you use it in. When they are in season, I use the white asparagus.

If you are going to make a stir fry, make a double recipe of asparagus and use the roasted asparagus in stir fry. Also, may be added to any of my vegetable soups.

Ratatouille (Summer Vegetable Ragout)

PER SERVING	
Calories	67
Fat	3 g.
Saturated Fat	0 g
Sodium	9 mg.
Sugar	5 g.
Carbohydrate	11 g.
Fiber	5 g.
Protein	2 g.

Prep Time: 20 minutes
Cook Time: 1 hour
Level: Easy
Serves 6

This is a classic and may be served warm or cold.

Ingredients

- 1 Japanese eggplant, sliced into rounds of about ⅜ inch
- 1 zucchini, sliced into rounds of about ⅜ inch
- 1 yellow onion, large dice or long thin slices
- 1 or 2 cloves garlic, sliced thinly
- 1 red bell pepper, sliced into half inch squares
- 2 diced tomatoes and a small can of tomato sauce or 1 15 oz. can diced tomatoes
- Handful of fresh parsley, chopped
- A few leaves of fresh basil, chopped
- Salt and white pepper to taste
- Olive oil or canola oil for sauté of veggies

Directions

Preheat the oven to 350 degrees.

Cut all the vegetables into pieces that will allow them to cook at the same rate in the oven.

Saute the veggies one at a time in a tablespoon of olive oil, adding oil or broth if needed to the eggplant to get the light caramelization.

Add each component of the dish to a 9 x 9 baking dish as they are completed. Add the tomatoes or tomato sauce. Cover with foil and cook in the oven for an hour, until the vegetables are tender. Then add the fresh parsley. Basil if you like.

This dish is the essence of summer vegetables. May be served with a soup, as a side dish. Or with a protein, such as a piece of baked or steamed fish and a carb, such as mashed potatoes, to make a meal.

It purées beautifully because of the sauce. It also freezes beautifully. It is well worth the effort of chopping the veggies.

For the Purée

Allow the dish to cool.

Take one cup of the vegetable ragout with an extra spoonful of sauce.

Place in the bowl of a mini food processor or the small pitcher of a blender.

Pulse five times to break up the vegetables.

Purée until smooth, adding sauce as needed.

Use a pump or a scoop of instant thickener to bind the purée.

Spinach Sauté

Prep Time: 10 minutes
Cook Time: 10 minutes
Level: Easy
Serves 4

PER SERVING

Calories	67
Fat	4 g.
Saturated Fat	1 g.
Sodium	106 mg.
Sugar	0 g.
Carbohydrate	5 g.
Fiber	2 g.
Protein	4 g.

Ingredients

- 1 bunch baby spinach or regular spinach in season
- 1 tablespoon olive oil
- 1 teaspoon lemon juice
- 1 small shallot, sliced thinly (optional)
- 1 clove garlic, sliced thinly (optional)
- 2 tablespoons grated parmesan cheese
- Water for purée

Directions

In a 12 inch skillet, heat up the olive oil on medium high heat and sauté the shallots until they are translucent, about a minute. (You can use any type of onion, including white onion or red onion or yellow onion, but shallots are sweet and add a wonderful flavor.)

Add garlic and sauté for a minute. Add the spinach and swirl to cover with the flavored oil. Add the lemon juice and a shot of lower sodium soy sauce. When spinach wilts, add the parmesan and let it melt.

For the Purée

Add the mixture to your blender, mini food processor or extractor and purée until you get the desired uniform smooth consistency. Add water or broth a tablespoon at a time to get the desired consistency. Use half a scoop or half a pump of instant thickener to bind the dish for service. This freezes beautifully.

Note: Leafy greens are nutrient dense. You can use bagged spinach, or bunch spinach. Make sure to wash thoroughly. You can also use frozen chopped spinach. This recipe can also be the base for a quiche or for an omelette using soft scrambled eggs.

You can also make this recipe using chard, rainbow chard or kale, if you remove the stems first.

Tip: You cannot exaggerate the importance of greens. This is a terrific way of incorporating them into the diet. It is too difficult to purée a green salad, so I use cooked greens. You can sauté a pack of baby spinach with a little garlic and pres the excess liquid out of it with a masher and a sieve, and purée the spinach with mashed potatoes for green potatoes. A treat for the eyes.

Braised Greens: Chard, Kale, Beets, Mustard Greens

Prep Time: 10 minutes
Cook Time: 30 minutes
Level: Easy
Serves 4

Greens are all the rage in the culinary world and with good reason. They are the great achievement of nature and a treasure house of nutrients.

Ingredients

- 1 bunch of greens, chard, kale, beet or mustard greens or combination
- 1 small onion diced, or 2 small shallots
- 2 tbsp. vegetable oil
- Broth to cover, either chicken or vegetarian, or plain water

Directions

Remove veins and stalks from greens. Slice greens into ribbons.

Sauté the onion or shallot in a 3 quart soup pot, add the greens and stir fry for a minute or two. Add the broth and cover with the lid slightly off center to allow steam to escape. Cook on low heat for twenty minutes, until greens are tender. Trimmed greens may also be cooked in an electric pressure cooker. This takes less time. The greens become very tender. Follow the manufacturer's direction as to the cooking time.

The electric pressure cooker is ideal for the quick cooking of collard greens. This is a favorite item of the soul food kitchen. Collards normally take a long time because they can be tough. Manufacturers' instructions provide times and amounts and types of liquid. Ham hock may be added for traditional soul food recipes.

For the Purée

Place cooked greens in a bowl. Allow the greens to cool. Add the cooked greens to the pitcher of a blander. Add the broth.

Purée, using the broth. If you are left with extra broth, add it to a homemade soup. Don't waste it, as it is full of precious phytochemicals.

To stabilize the vegetable purée, use a half pump or a half scoop of instant thickener. Combine thoroughly.

This veggie freezes well and can be added to soup.

Variation

The classic Italian soup made of greens is made with escarole. Sauté a clove of garlic in a tablespoon of olive oil, adding a bunch of escarole that has been trimmed of stems and veins, and covering with chicken broth and simmering until tender. This is a delicious and nutritious soup.

When the soup has cooled, add it to the pitcher of a blender.

Purée until completely smooth.

Thicken with a pump or a scoop of instant thickener per eight ounces of soup, until the soup is the correct consistency for the swallow. Adjust thickener as needed as no two locations have the same climate.

Note: You cannot exaggerate the importance of greens. Add cooked, puréed greens to soups and sauces.

Here is an idea for a festive holiday side dish. Stir fry a pack of baby spinach in a tablespoon or two of olive oil. Add a squeeze of Gourmet Garden garlic paste. It is already a paste, a quickie ingredient. Or use one finely minced garlic clove.

When the spinach is wilted, allow it to cool.

Stir the spinach purée into a one-cup serving of mashed potatoes and you have green potatoes. One of the great problems in the dysphagia kitchen is patient boredom. This is a way of creating pleasing color on the plate. We eat with our eyes. We use our other senses to make up for the swallowing disorder. Try it at Christmas or St. Patrick's Day. Try it at the beginning of Spring.

Broccoli Parmesan

Prep Time: 10 minutes
Cook Time: 20 minutes
Level: Easy
Serves 4

Calories	119
Fat	11 g.
Saturated Fat	2 g.
Sodium	54 mg.
Sugar	0 g.
Carbohydrate	4 g.
Fiber	0 g.
Protein	3 g.

Ingredients

- 1 head broccoli, cut into florets
- 1 clove garlic, sliced thinly
- 3 tablespoons olive oil
- 2 tbsp. fresh lemon juice
- 2 tablespoons parmesan cheese
- Water for purée

Directions

Steam the broccoli by your favorite method until tender.

In a 12-inch skillet, heat up the olive oil and sauté the garlic for a minute on medium high heat. Add the broccoli and swirl to cover with the garlic-y oil. Add the lemon juice and the parmesan, and swirl in pan until cheese melts. Done.

For the Purée

Purée, adding water until you get the desired uniform smooth consistency. This freezes beautifully.

Tip: I keep my kitchen tools simple, but some small kitchen appliances are excellent for the purée chef. To all those who wish to simplify tasks in the dysphagia kitchen: For reviews of the newer appliances, please go to the Essential Purée website.

Tip: In the time-honored chef's tradition of using everything and wasting nothing, I save the stalks of the broccoli and peel them and steam them. They are excellent in vegetable soups, such as minestrone, or make a delicious broccoli soup when puréed with chicken stock. The flavor is terrific and the nutritional benefits are excellent.

Brussel Sprouts with Shallots

PER SERVING

Calories	99
Fat	7 g.
Saturated Fat	1 g.
Sodium	9 mg.
Sugar	0 g.
Carbohydrate	8 g.
Fiber	3 g.
Protein	3 g.

Prep Time: 12 minutes
Cook Time: 40 minutes
Level: Easy
Serves 4

My mother adored Brussels sprouts and these alternative recipes were developed for her.

Ingredients

- 1 pound Brussels sprouts, with the cores trimmed
- 2 shallots, peeled and sliced thinly
- 2 tbsp. olive oil
- Salt and white pepper

Directions

Preheat oven to 375 degrees

Trim the Brussel sprouts and cut them in half.

Trim and cut the shallots into slices.

In a bowl, combine the olive oil, salt and white pepper.

Mix in the Brussels sprouts and the shallots. Add a clove or two of garlic, if you like.

Roast the Brussel sprouts in the oven for forty minutes, until tender and only slightly caramelized.

For the Purée

When the veggies have cooled, place one cup plus several tablespoons of water or broth into the bowl of a mini food processor or the small pitcher of a blender.

Pulse a few times to break down the vegetable.

Purée to get a smooth texture.

To bind the vegetable, add a half scoop or a half pump of instant thickener

Tip: Excessive browning may result in sharp pieces in purée. Avoid this or remove any brown dried bits before purée.

Tip: Alternate methods of cooking this fantastic veggie: Steam the sprouts. You can even boil them in a shallow amount of water, using the juice of half a lemon to flavor the water.

Cabbage Sauté

Prep Time: 10 minutes
Cook Time: 20 minutes
Level: Easy
Serves 4

PER SERVING

Calories	66
Fat	7 g.
Saturated Fat	1 g.
Sodium	1 mg.
Sugar	1 g.
Carbohydrate	1 g.
Fiber	0 g.
Protein	0 g.

Ingredients

- Half a head of cabbage, of any variety, cored and sliced about a pound
- Half an onion, sliced thinly
- 2 tbsp. vegetable oil
- Optional: 1 Golden Delicious apple, peeled and sliced into half moons

Directions

Cabbage should be sliced thinly.

Brown the onions in half the oil until golden. Add the rest of the oil and stir in and wilt the cabbage. Stir fry until the cabbage reduces in size and is mixed in well with the onion. Add several tablespoons water and continue cooking. This is a great side dish for beef or pork.

For the Purée

Allow the dish to cool.

Take one cup of the cabbage and a few tablespoons of the cooking liquid and place in the bowl of a mini food processor or the small pitcher of a blender.

Pulse five times to break down the veggie.

Purée until smooth. Or purée in a nutrition extractor such as a NutriBullet for twenty seconds

Bind with a half pump or a half scoop of instant thickener.

If you wish, sauté an apple, such as a Golden Delicious, with the cabbage. Apple will cook down and add a sweetness to the veggie.

Roasted Cauliflower: Adventures in Florets

Calories	66
Fat	4 g.
Saturated Fat	0 g.
Sodium	43 mg.
Sugar	3 g.
Carbohydrate	8 g.
Fiber	4 g.
Protein	3 g.

Prep Time: 10 minutes
Cook Time: 45 minutes
Level: Easy

Ingredients

- 1 head cauliflower
- Olive oil
- Salt and white pepper

Directions

Preheat oven to 400 degrees.

Cut cauliflower in half and remove the core. Cut into florets of the same size.

In a large bowl, mix olive oil, salt and white pepper with cauliflower florets

On a sheet pan, roast in oven for forty minutes until tender. Cauliflower should be golden, but not caramelized as this will lead to bits in purée which will be hard to swallow.

When the dish cools, add a cup of the florets to the bowl of a mini food processor or the pitcher of a blender.

For the Purée

Purée with water. A number of good chefs recommend water as a cooking liquid, although any broth, such as chicken broth or vegetable broth may be used. If one likes creamed cauliflower, add a heaping tablespoon of lower fat sour cream.

To bind the dish, add a half scoop or a half pump of instant thickener.

When puréed, this vegetable has a distinctive nutty flavor gained from roasting.

Cauliflower, Cruciform Extraordinaire

PER SERVING

Calories	126
Fat	4.5 g.
Saturated Fat	1.5 g.
Sodium	543 mg.
Sugar	11 g.
Carbohydrate	18 g.
Fiber	5 g.
Protein	5 g.

Prep Time: 10 minutes
Cook Time: 12 minutes
Level: Easy
Serves 4

If you do not know cauliflower, here's your chance to get to know the amazing superfood.

Ingredients
- 1 head cauliflower, cored and cut into florets, about a pound
- 1 jar Ethnic Gourmet Calcutta Masala simmer sauce

Directions

Steam the cauliflower until tender. I use a three-tiered steam-injected steamer, a small kitchen appliance commercially available, but any steamer will do, including the lotus-shaped steamer that inserts in the bottom of a stock pot, with water underneath. If you use this last method, please cover the pot to keep the steam in.

When I use the lotus steamer, I put the cauliflower in whole and break it into florets after it is cooked. When I use the electric steamer, I slice the cauliflower into florets. I set the timer for twelve minutes and judge for doneness.

When using the lotus shaped steamer in a stock pot, I test with a knife to see if the cauliflower is tender, approximately twenty minutes. Be careful of escaping steam.

If cauliflower is tender, I turn off the heat and wait a few moments, then open the pot, being careful not to get steam burns.

Add half the jar of simmer sauce to a fry pan and warm it. Add the cauliflower, coating it well.

Tip: I use a high quality commercially prepared simmer sauce as a shortcut. Sometimes one simply has to get food on the table. This sauce does not have a lot of heat, but it has a lot of flavor. This is the Ethnic Gourmet Calcutta Masala. It is mild. You can add a tablespoon of yogurt to the sauce to enrich and thicken. You can add a half teaspoon of a favorite chutney if the chutney is smooth. This adds to the flavor.

Healthy Cooking Methods

You can make the curried cauliflower using the stir fry method.

Stir fry is an excellent method of cooking, as it is quick and imparts flavor. Heat a tablespoon of good oil over medium high heat and drop in the florets. Stir frying for two minutes, then add steaming liquid, such as water or broth or curry sauce, cover and lower the heat. Simmer for 10 minutes over low heat until cauliflower is tender.

My own curry sauce is made from Thai curry paste and coconut milk, unsweetened variety, and light. Sit fry or steam the cauliflower and finish in the curry sauce until tender, approximately fifteen minutes over low heat. Use a 15 oz. can of lite coconut milk and a tablespoon of Thai Curry Paste, red.

For the Purée

When the dish cools, take a cup of the vegetable and add it to the bowl of a mini food processor or the small pitcher of a blender.

Pulse five times to break up the cauliflower. Add a tablespoon of plain yogurt, low fat if desired. Add a half teaspoon of a smooth chutney, if desired.

Purée until smooth.

Bind the purée with a half pump or a half scoop of instant thickener.

Variation

Lemon Butter. In my opinion, simple is better. You can never go wrong with the classic flavor profile of lemon and butter. Take 2 tbsp. of lemon juice and add to 2 tablespoons melted butter or non-transfat margarine and coat the cauliflower with the sauce before purée.

Assembling the Meal

This cauliflower pairs well with a piece of fish and mashed potato and braised greens on the side.

Garlic Green Beans

Prep Time: 10 minutes
Cook Time: 18 minutes
Level: Easy
Serves 4

Calories	154
Fat	11 g.
Saturated Fat	2 g.
Sodium	130 mg.
Sugar	2 g.
Carbohydrate	14 g.
Fiber	4 g.
Protein	3 g.

Ingredients

- 1 lb. green beans
- 2 cloves garlic
- 3 tablespoons olive oil
- 1 tablespoon lemon juice
- 2 large tablespoons Italian bread crumbs
- Sprinkle of parmesan cheese

Directions

Trim string beans of ends and strings. Steam to softness, but with beans still retaining color. I use a three-tiered vegetable steamer where each tier has one layer of beans and all beans steam evenly. For years, I used a folding steamer that fits inside a larger pot.

Remove beans from steamer. You may plunge the beans into an ice bath if you wish to set the color. This is a bowl filled with ice and water. Use a mesh sieve.

In a sauté pan, place thinly sliced garlic and allow to cook for one minute, until slightly soft, but not browned.

Add beans to pan and swirl in garlic oil. Add lemon juice to taste. I like lemony beans, so I use more. Add bread crumbs and parmesan cheese to make a sauce.

For the Purée

Allow beans to cool. Place a cup of beans and several tablespoons of water or broth into the bowl of a mini food processor or the pitcher of a blender.

Pulse five times to break up the beans.

Purée until smooth, adding water or broth if necessary.

Bind the purée with a half scoop or a half pump of instant thickener.

Ginger Carrots

Prep Time: 5 minutes
Cook Time: 10 minutes
Level: Easy
Serves 4

Ingredients

- 4 carrots, peeled and sliced into half moons (or 1 cup baby carrots, peeled, in package in the grocery store)
- 2 tbsp. vegetable oil or unsalted butter
- 1 tbsp. sliced fresh ginger, matchsticks about an inch long
- 1 tbsp. honey

Directions

Steam the carrots for twelve minutes until they are tender.

In a skillet, over medium high heat, melt the butter or heat the vegetable oil. Stir in the ginger and allow to become aromatic, cooking for a minute. Add the honey and allow to mix in for about thirty seconds. This is your ginger glaze.

Swirl carrots in the ginger glaze. Add vegetables and slowly stir, allowing glaze to coat the carrots.

For the Purée

Allow the carrots to cool.

Place one cup of carrots In the bowl of a mini food processor or the small pitcher of a blender.

Add several tablespoons of broth, water or carrot juice.

Pulse five times to break the carrots up. Purée until smooth.

Use a half pump or a half scoop of instant thickener to bind the dish..

 Tip: For steaming, I use a three-tiered steamer. The only rule: Don't crowd the veggies.

Variation

For a deeper flavor, add to the sauté pan 1 tbsp. of hoisin sauce from the Asian market or Asian section of the grocery store.

This sauce is made from plums and adds a depth of flavor and saltiness to the dish.

It also makes an excellent change from the usual, carrots with a plain butter sauce. Don't overcook the hoisin. Allow it to merely warm and coat the veggies before the purée.

Whole Grains

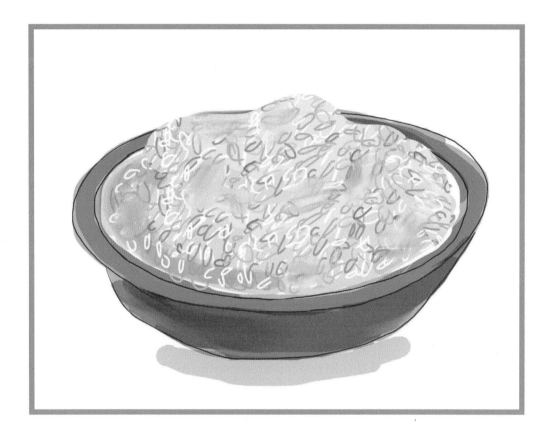

The importance of whole grains in the diet cannot be overestimated. They are recommended as heart-healthy by the American Heart Association and as healthy for diabetics by the American Diabetic Association. They metabolize slowly and do not spike blood sugar, therefore do not produce a spike in insulin.

The best cooking method for rendering the grains tender for the purée is to cook them in an electric pressure cooker or a mini rice cooker. The outer coat of the grain softens enough for a smooth purée. You get the benefits of superior nutrients and also get the fiber. For the patient with swallowing difficulties, the investment in the appliance is well worth it.

Rice

Yield: 8 half-cup servings

Calories	175
Fat	0 g.
Saturated Fat	0 g.
Sodium	1 mg.
Sugar	0 g.
Carbohydrate	38 g.
Fiber	1 g.
Protein	4 g.

Ingredients

- 2 cups rice (for purée, I like brown basmati rice)
- 4½ cups water
- Pinch salt

Directions

The general rule for rice is two to one, water to rice. For basmati rice, the ratio is 2 and ¼ cups to one cup rice.

I measure out my rice into a large mixing bowl and wash it several times and drain it until the water runs clear. The great cooks of the Zen Buddhist tradition in Japan advise taking care with your rice, because it becomes your eyes. I also look for any green kernels or any little stones.

I then measure the rice into the pot, add the salt for softening of the grain, and the water, close the pot and let it go. I check on the cooking about halfway through.

Tip: I always make extra rice to have it on hand for puréeing it with a protein, for making my Chinese fried rice, or for making rice pudding, which my mother loves. Because my mother is a pulmonary patient, I try to limit the amount of dairy that she eats. I have tried making rice pudding with non-dairy milks, such as soy milk and almond milk, but the only non-dairy milk that works for this is light coconut milk.

Tip: With a nod to the American chef Ming Tsai, who grew up in his parents Chinese restaurant. The best way to get a fluffy fried rice is to freeze cooked rice, either on a sheet pan in a single layer and then store in a zip-lock bag or directly in a single layer in the zip-loc. I estimate the mount of rice that I will need for four servings of fried rice, approximately two cups of cooked rice.

I freeze rice in individual zipped bags, dating it for use within 30 days. The kernels dry out a little bit in the freezing. This is perfect for fried rice and yields an excellent texture when combined with sautéed veggies and protein, a little stock and a little lower sodium soy.

Tip: Rice is also an ingredient in my salmon in puff pastry. For this dish, one wants hydrated rice, not dry rice. I saute a little onion or shallot, and stir fry the rice with a tablespoon of oil and a couple of tablespoons of water or chicken broth or vegetable broth and a shot of soy sauce. This gives the rice a soft texture for the purée.

Quinoa

Prep Time: 1 minute
Cook Time: 15 minutes
Level: Easy
Serves 4

PER SERVING

Calories	156
Fat	3 g.
Saturated Fat	0 g.
Sodium	2 mg.
Sugar	0 g.
Carbohydrate	27 g.
Fiber	3 g.
Protein	6 g.

Quinoa (pronounced keen-wa) is a high protein grain originally from South America. It can be a little boring all by itself. I add a little onion and garlic.

For festive occasions, add a couple of tablespoons of smooth walnut butter or smooth almond butter and a handful of dried cranberries soaked in water or broth for 5 minutes to rehydrate. You don't want dry ingredients for patients who have swallowing difficulties.

Ingredients

- 1 cup quinoa, rinsed in clear water 2 cups water
- Shake of salt

Directions

Rinse your quinoa well in a strainer before using. This eliminates any bitterness in taste.

Equipment: For the dysphagia kitchen, it is important to render whole grains to a soft texture that is easy to purée. Use an electric pressure cooker or the turboconvection cooker. Use the times recommended in the manufacturer's directions.

For the Purée

When the grain has cooled, take one cup of the grain and ¼ cup of broth and add to the bowl of a mini food processor or the small pitcher of a blender.

Pulse five times to break down the grain. Purée until smooth.

May be puréed with several tablespoons of smooth gravy. May also be puréed with several tablespoons of soup, either cream or broth based.

Kasha or Buckwheat Groats

Calories	175
Fat	0 g.
Saturated Fat	0 g.
Sodium	1 mg.
Sugar	0 g.
Carbohydrate	38 g.
Fiber	1 g.
Protein	4 g.

Prep Time: 10 minutes
Cook Time: 20 minutes
Level: Easy
Yield: 4 half cup servings

Kasha has a delicious nutty flavor and can become a favorite. Buckwheat is a nutrition powerhouse. This is a heavier grain, and I use it mostly in the winter, to accompany any protein such as beef or lamb, or even seafood. In the summer, it can be served cold with salad ingredients such as avocado and tomato. Use it like faro or bulgur wheat.

Ingredients

- 1 cup kasha, fine mill
- 1 medium onion, cut into fine slivers
- 1 carrot cut into half moon slices, thin
- 1 clove garlic, sliced thinly
- 2 cups chicken broth
- Soy sauce to taste
- Salt and white pepper to taste

Directions

Pan toast the kasha in a dry cast iron skillet for depth of flavor. Remove from skillet.

Sauté diced onion in a tablespoon of vegetable oil, until translucent. Add the carrot and sauté for two minutes, garlic goes in at the last minute.

Add the buckwheat, add the chicken broth and soy sauce. Bring to the boil and lower heat to a simmer. Set a cover slightly off the pan to allow the steam to escape. Cook for twenty minutes, until kasha is soft.

If liquid becomes too low, add more. Can also be made with vegetable stock or with water. I made it this way for my dad. Because of the fine mill of the kasha, this cooks up very tender. Do not let it go so far that it turns to mush, unless you wish to serve it as a porridge.

For the Purée

When the kasha has cooled, take one cup of the kasha and veggies and one half cup of chicken broth.

Pulse four times to combine. Purée until smooth. Add a pump or a scoop of instant thickener to bind the purée. Combine thoroughly.

Since it is difficult to purée lettuce or any other green in a summer salad, in summer I add my greens to soups and sauces. In winter, the braised greens can be puréed with whole grains.

For those on gluten free diets, use kasha instead of bulgur wheat.

Freeze extra portions in individual storage containers to use in soups and as a side dish with a protein.

Tip: This can also be added to a warm winter salad of braised greens with roasted mushrooms and a chopped tomato with vinaigrette dressing. Purées beautifully.

Breakfast

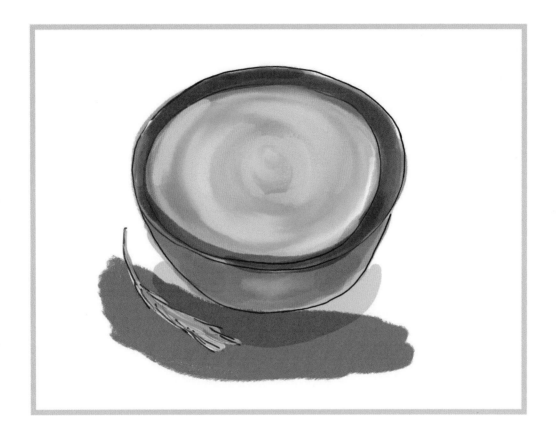

Light Lunch
Salads and Soups

Steel-Cut Oatmeal with Yogurt & Honey

PER SERVING

Calories	351
Fat	4 g.
Saturated Fat	1 g.
Sodium	68 mg.
Sugar	50 g.
Carbohydrate	76 g.
Fiber	6 g.
Protein	8 g.

Prep Time: 5 minutes
Cook Time: As on package
Level: Easy
Serves 1

My mother loved oatmeal for breakfast. Steel-cut oats are less processed and have more nutrients than the more commercial versions of rolled oats. The final product has less sugar and more fiber.

Equipment: To render oatmeal soft and tender for the purée, use the Wolfgang Puck mini rice cooker, the Ming Tsai turboconvection cooker or an electric pressure cooker.

Ingredients

- ¼ cup steel cut oatmeal, 5 minute variety
- 1 cup water
- 1 dash salt
- ½ cup milk
- ¼ cup Greek yogurt
- 1 tsp good local honey

Directions

Following package directions, add the oats to the water and salt. I add a shake of cinnamon.

Turn on rice cooker and allow it to go through its cycle, stirring occasionally. This is about five minutes. Oatmeal should be soft and tender. If it needs more time, close the cooker and turn on cook cycle. Check every minute. Be mindful of steam.

Follow manufacturers' instructions for pressure cooker or turbo convection cooker.

For the Purée

When oatmeal cools, add one cup to the bowl of a mini food processor or the small cup of a blender. Add milk, honey or sweetener of choice, and yogurt.

Pulse five times then purée until smooth.

Check with your healthcare provider to see if you can include any of the following: Puréed fruit. Dried goji berries will rehydrate in any of the cookers and will become soft for the purée. Puréed banana will boost the nutrients. Raw wheat germ is soft and a nutritional powerhouse.

Blintzes with Blueberry Sauce and Sour Cream

PER SERVING

Calories	323
Fat	3 g.
Saturated Fat	1 g.
Sodium	282 mg.
Sugar	35 g.
Carbohydrate	63 g.
Fiber	2 g.
Protein	11 g.

Prep Time: 5 minutes
Cook Time: 16 minutes
Level: Easy
Yield: 1 serving is 2 blintzes with 2 tbsp. low fat sour cream and ¼ cup blueberry sauce

This is a family favorite from the old days of eating breakfast out on Sunday on Miami Beach in the great old time restaurants, Wolfie's on Lincoln Road or Junior's on Collins Avenue.

Ingredients

- Package of Ratner's Cheese Blintzes
- Blueberry Sauce (see recipe)
- Low fat sour cream

Directions

Either defrost the blintzes and brown on each side for four minutes in a little butter or non trans-fat margarine or paint the frozen blintzes with vegetable oil and bake on a sheet pan lined with parchment for eight minutes on a side.

Top each blintz with a generous teaspoon of blueberry sauce and a dollop of sour cream. Makes an excellent purée and an excellent Sunday breakfast. The meal is sweet.

For the Purée

When blintzes have cooled, break up one or two in the bowl of a mini food processor. Add a generous teaspoon of puréed blueberry sauce and a tablespoon of sour cream for each blintz.

Pulse five times to break up and incorporate. Purée until smooth, about 10 seconds.

If I am time-challenged, this is one of my go-to convenience foods. I keep them in my freezer.

Tip: Whenever you purée a dish with ricotta cheese, the volume increases because of the air. What is a normal serving of three blintzes increases in volume and looks like a larger serving. The food is light in taste and texture as a result, but is the same nutritionally and in terms of calories.

Blueberry Sauce for Pancakes, Oatmeal, Blintzes, Shortcake or Ice Cream

PER SERVING

Calories	123
Fat	0 g.
Saturated Fat	0 g.
Sodium	2 mg.
Sugar	25 g.
Carbohydrate	29 g.
Fiber	2 g.
Protein	1 g.

Prep Time: 5 minutes
Cook Time: 20 minutes
Level: Easy
Yield: 4 half-cup servings

Any homemade fruit sauce is more delicious and nutritious than the flavored syrups for pancakes you can buy pre-bottled. This sauce has the added virtue of flexibility—add it to oatmeal or any other hot cereal or to ice cream for a nutrition boost.

Equipment: Nutrition extractor such as a NutriBullet or a NutriNinja.

Ingredients

- 1 pint blueberries, washed, drained and dried on a paper towel
- 1 cup water
- 2 tbsp. fresh lemon juice
- ¼ cup maple syrup or honey or agave syrup
- 2 tbsp. corn starch dissolved in two tablespoons water, a slurry for thickening

Directions

Using a nutrition extractor, place a pint of blueberries and a cup of water in the small cup of a nutrition extractor.

Extract the fruit and water in 10 second increments until the fruit is liquefied.

Run the liquefied fruit through a mesh sieve lined with cheesecloth using a silicone spatula. This should remove any particles of skin or fiber and give you a smooth liquid fruit for making the sauce.

Place liquefied blueberries in saucepan and add water. Bring to boil and reduce heat to simmer. Add lemon juice and sweetener.

Allow to simmer gently for five minutes to cook the fruit.

Add corn starch slurry and stir. Mixture will thicken as it boils. Keep an eye on it. Cook for two minutes until raw taste of cornstarch disappears.

Allow sauce to cool in pan for 10 minutes and then purée. I put half in the fridge for use during the week and freeze half for use during the month.

If you use the nutrition extractor, it is possible to make sauces from other fruits, either fresh or frozen.

The nutrition extractor will liquefy blackberries, raspberries or even strawberries. It will also liquefy fresh mangoes, when the flesh is cut from the pit, eliminating any strands.

Before cooking, select your fruit, whether frozen or fresh.

Place a cup or two of the fruit in the small cup of a nutrition extractor.

Extract in increments of 10 seconds to liquefy.

Run the liquefied fruit through a mesh sieve with a lining of cheesecloth, using a silicone spatula to put the fruit through the sieve. This step eliminates fibers, skin and seeds in the fruit product.

Remove the liquefied fruit from the cup and place in a saucepan.

Cook the liquefied fruit according to the instructions in the recipe for the blueberry sauce.

Hint: Quickie Alternative to Fruit Sauce

As a go to convenience ingredient, use seedless raspberry, blackberry or strawberry jam. There are a number of good products available commercially.

Use a teaspoon of the product in the purée of the blintz as a substitute for the fresh fruit sauce. May also be made from blackberries, raspberries or strawberries.

In the winter, I use frozen organic strawberries which I buy and stock up on when on sale in whole foods store. Recipe may be doubled.

Scrambled Eggs and Mashed Potatoes

PER SERVING

Calories	221
Fat	10 g.
Saturated Fat	3 g.
Sodium	147 mg.
Sugar	2 g.
Carbohydrate	19 g.
Fiber	2 g.
Protein	15 g.

Prep Time: 5 minutes
Cook Time: 10 minutes
Level: Easy
Serves 1

I found that it was difficult to purée home fries for a classic American accompaniment to breakfast, because there were hard particles in the purée. The mashed potatoes deliver flavor and are a good substitute for home fries.

Ingredients

- 1 pat butter or non trans-fat margarine such as Smart Balance
- 2 or 3 eggs, lightly beaten
- 2 tablespoon of milk
- ½ cup serving of homemade mashed potatoes, warmed

Directions

Melt butter in skillet. Scramble eggs softly in pan.

Warm the ½ cup serving of mashed potatoes.

For Service

The eggs should be of a custard consistency. The mashed potatoes should be of a custard consistence when prepared according to the recipe. Place eggs in one dish and potatoes in a second dish and alternate bites for service.

Tip: To create a classic American breakfast, I add two chicken and apple sausages. I use the Applegate Naturals brand. These are lower in fat and sodium than standard breakfast sausages. Warmed them for 4 minutes per side in a pan, until heated through. Purée until smooth in the small bowl of a mini food processor.

Buckwheat Pancakes with Homemade Blueberry Sauce

Calories	184
Fat	7 g.
Saturated Fat	1 g.
Sodium	403 mg.
Sugar	6 g.
Carbohydrate	18 g.
Fiber	2 g.
Protein	12 g.

Calories	254
Fat	12 g.
Saturated Fat	3 g.
Sodium	473 mg.
Sugar	6 g.
Carbohydrate	18 g.
Fiber	2 g.
Protein	18 g.

Prep Time: 15 minutes
Cook Time: 15 minutes
Level: Easy
Yield: 12 silver dollar size pancakes of about three inches in diameter

This was Mom's classic Sunday breakfast.

Equipment: Electric griddle for pancakes. Steaming rack of mini rice cooker for the egg. Or the steaming rack of a multi-cooker. Or the bottom tier of the three-tiered steamer.

Ingredients

- ⅔ cup buckwheat pancake mix
- 2 tbsp. vegetable oil
- 1 egg, beaten lightly
- 1 cup milk
- Splash of good vanilla extract
- Splash of local honey

Directions

Stir ingredients lightly but do not over mix. Heat griddle to 375 degrees. I use a small gravy ladle to make uniform silver dollar pancakes.

In a dish sprayed with cooking spray, lightly steam an egg in the steaming rack of your mini rice cooker or any other steaming device.

The egg should be soft. This means two minutes or two and a half minutes to a coddled or soft boiled texture. Egg should not contain hard whites. Yolk should be soft and runny. Place a pat of butter in with the egg, if you like.

In the microwave, heat one tablespoon butter or margarine—I use the non-trans-fat Smart Balance—and two tablespoons real maple syrup on 30 seconds at 50 per cent power.

For the Purée

This purées nicely. If I need extra liquid to get the desired consistency, I use a little water or a little more blueberry sauce.

In the bowl of a mini food processor or the small pitcher of a blender with double blades, break up 3 of the silver dollar pancakes

Add the steamed egg to the bowl of the mini food processor or the small pitcher of the blender.

Add 2 tbsp. melted butter or non trans fat margarine such as Smart Balance.

Add 4 tbsp. good maple syrup.

Add 4 tbsp. puréed blueberry sauce.

Pulse five times to combine all the elements. Use water or blueberry sauce if purée is too stiff.

Purée for 10 seconds until all elements are incorporated into the purée.

Can be served with Applegate Naturals Chicken and Apple Sausage puréed into the dish. This brand has no saturated fat.

If desired, warm three of the chicken and apple sausages according to the directions on the package. When they are cool, they may be broken up and added to the bowl of the mini food processor before the pancakes are added.

Pulse five times to break up the sausages. They will purée to a smooth texture when the liquids are added.

Tip: I use Arrowhead Mills Organic Buckwheat Pancake and Waffle Mix from a whole foods store. I store it in a plastic bag in the refrigerator to keep the grains fresh. I make one recipe of pancakes as listed on the package, but I doctor the recipe, adding a little vanilla and honey to sweeten it.

Tip: When mixing up a batter of pancakes, why not griddle the entire batch of pancakes? Extra pancakes from the recipe are stored in a good zippered freezer bag and dated. They freeze well and make two or three more breakfasts.

Split Pea Soup

Prep Time: 10 minutes
Cook Time: 1 hour
Level: Easy
Serves 4

PER SERVING

Calories	190
Fat	4 g.
Saturated Fat	4 g.
Sodium	676 mg
Sugar	5 g.
Carbohydrate	27 g.
Fiber	9 g.
Protein	13 g.

This was Cathie G's favorite soup. I like the vegetarian version, but if you choose, instead of using the cumin, you can flavor your soup with a ham hock

Ingredients

- ¾ cup split peas
- ¼ cup French lentils, soaked in a cup of water overnight
- 1 medium yellow onion, diced
- 2 carrots, halved and sliced in half moons
- 1 clove garlic, sliced
- 1 tbsp. olive oil or vegetable oil
- ½ tsp cumin
- 1 tbsp. lower sodium soy sauce
- ¼ teaspoon dried thyme
- 1 quart lower sodium chicken stock. Alternatively, water to cover plus one inch more

Directions

Rinse peas in bowl of water and drain once or twice until water runs clear. Do the same for the lentils. Soak peas for at least an hour in clear water to rehydrate them. Soak lentils overnight. Drain peas and lentils.

Over medium high heat, saute onion until translucent, about one minute. Add carrot, and sauté for an additional minute, add garlic and saute one minute.

Add the cumin, the thyme and the soy sauce and cook for about thirty seconds. Our family prefers a soup without ham hocks and this step cooks out the rawness in the cumin. Cumin is a smoky spice and imparts that depth of flavor that some people like from the ham hock. If your family likes the ham, by all means, add it here.

Add peas and lentils and cover with stock. A trick I use is the vegetable bouillon cube that contains herbs. I use the Rapunzel brand that I buy at the whole foods store, one that does not contain sea salt. This is a high quality product.

Bring soup to boil over medium high heat. Lower and simmer for one hour. After five minutes, a foam will form on top of the soup. This is caused by impurities in the vegetables coming to the surface. Please skim foam.

Sometimes the peas absorb liquid. If so, add more water or stock. Cook until peas are soft. Adjust seasoning. The lower sodium soy sauce also adds a depth of flavor that compares very well with adding ham.

For the Purée

Allow soup to cool.

Add a cup of soup to the bowl of a mini food processor or a blender.

Purée until smooth, about twenty seconds.

Divide the pot of soup into individual portions, label and freeze. This is batch cooking. You have three extra servings for a quickie meal or snack.

Note: If you try to purée a hot liquid and do not vent the blender or the Ninja, the soup will expand and go all over the place. So do not purée a very hot liquid. Freezes very well.

Tip: Peas can be soaked for several hours. Soak lentils overnight. I buy organic peas at the whole foods store because they are fresher bought in bulk than the packaged ones bought in the supermarket and give a better texture. The price is about the same, with the bulk buy in the whole foods store equaling out to the packaging in the supermarket.

Matzo Ball Soup

Prep Time: 15 minutes
Cook Time: 20 minutes
Level: Intermediate
Serves 4

PER SERVING

Calories	202
Fat	9 g.
Saturated Fat	2 g.
Sodium	352 g
Sugar	4 g.
Carbohydrate	17 g.
Fiber	.5 g.
Protein	8 g.

My dad taught me how to make this soup. We asked our favorite deli owner how to make light matzo balls. He told us that if he revealed the secret, he would have to kill us, so we figured it out on our own. The secret is in the egg whites. It is labor intensive to make the matzo balls but delicious. Frozen matzo balls are now available in the international freezer section of the supermarket. These have not yet been tested in the Essential Purée kitchen.

Ingredients

The Matzo Balls

- ½ cup matzo meal
- 1 large egg, separated, white only
- 2 tablespoons vegetable oil
- 2 tablespoons chicken broth
- 2 tablespoons club soda at room temperature
- 1 tsp. Gourmet Garden parsley paste (optional)
- 2 quarts water for boiling matzo balls
- 1 quart chicken stock, your own or store bought(lower sodium) for soup

The Soup

- 1 qt. chicken broth
- 2 carrots, cut into sections
- 2 parsnips, cut into halves lengthwise and then into diagonal slices
- 1 teaspoon Gourmet Garden parsley paste
- 1 teaspoon Gourmet Garden dill paste
- ½ Vidalia onion
- 2 chicken breasts, skinless and boneless

Directions

Saute the onion until translucent, two minutes, adding the clove of garlic for the last minute, so it does not burn.

Add the carrot and sauté for two minutes.

Add zucchini and sauté for two minutes.

Add the diced tomato. If you like the flavor, you can buy diced tomato with garlic, basil and oregano in the market. If you buy plain diced tomato, at this point, add a pinch of dried oregano. Use a light touch, because oregano can overpower the dish.

Add the chicken broth and the pasta and cook for twenty minutes.

For the last several minutes, add a teaspoon of fresh parsley and basil, chopped finely.

Drain the beans and rinse them. Add the beans, stir and warm the beans for five minutes.

Purée and serve. The beans and pasta make for an excellent purée.

The Matzo Balls

Add the matzo meal, parsley and a pinch of salt to a bowl—I use a nonreactive stainless steel mixing bowl as the mixture will have to be chilled after mixing. My dad used to put pepper in the matzo balls as well, because he didn't like under-seasoned matzo balls.

Whip the egg white until frothy, about a minute. Hold to one side.

In a small bowl, combine the wet ingredients, the vegetable oil, the broth, the club soda. Add to dry ingredients with the egg white and mix well. Cover and put in the refrigerator for half an hour until well chilled.

Bring water to a gentle boil. I make one-inch matzo balls with my hands or with a one-inch cookie dropper or ice cream scoop. The secret here is gentle handling and a loose pack. Otherwise you will have matzo balls of stone.

Drop into water and cook for twenty minutes. Some people recommend cooking with a cover. I cook with an open pot. Remove from water with a spider when done. Cut one open and make sure it is cooked through.

The Soup:

Put chicken broth in a soup pot, bring to a boil, then turn down to a light simmer.

Add chicken, carrot, parsnip, onion and herbs and cook for fifteen minutes until chicken is done and the veggies are soft. Allow to cool. Remove chicken and cut into one inch cubes for purée. Remove onion and discard. Remove herbs.

For the Purée

In the small pitcher of a blender, place 4 ounces of the chicken breast.

Pulse five times to chop the chicken.

Break up two matzo balls and add to the pitcher. Add a quarter cup of broth.

Pulse five times to break up the matzo balls and broth and combine with the chicken.

Add a piece of carrot and a piece of parsnip and the rest of the broth.

Purée until smooth.

Tip: Quickie version: In the freezer section of my supermarket, I discovered frozen Matzo balls. The brand is Meal Mart. You drop the frozen Matzo balls in chicken soup and simmer for 20 minutes. You do not need to thaw them. Surprisingly good, especially when you have to get a meal on the table. Guilt-free matzo balls.

Minestrone

(Italian Vegetable Noodle Soup)

Prep Time: 10 minutes
Cook Time: 1 hour
Level: Easy
Serves 4

PER SERVING

Calories	199
Fat	1 g.
Saturated Fat	0 g.
Sodium	153 mg.
Sugar	1 g.
Carbohydrate	34 g.
Fiber	11 g.
Protein	16 g.

This version of the classic Italian vegetable noodle soup with beans is packed with nutrition and fiber.

Ingredients

- 1 medium yellow onion, sliced
- 1 clove garlic, sliced
- 1 carrot, sliced into half moons
- 1 zucchini, sliced into circles, then half moons
- 1 quart lower sodium chicken broth (or vegetable broth)
- 1 cup small shell pasta
- 1 can beans, either light kidney beans or white cannellini beans
- 1 can diced tomatoes, lower sodium. San Marzano tomatoes have depth of flavor. Squeeze the whole tomatoes in your hands over a bowl with a mesh sieve. This will catch any seeds. Add the tomatoes and the juice to the soup, or 1 ½ cups fresh plum tomatoes, seeded and chopped. Same method works. Mesh sieve over a bowl will catch the seeds. Use the chopped fresh tomato and the juice.

Directions

This is a terrific vegetable soup, so if you have leftover cooked string beans, for example, by all means, add them.

Saute the onion until translucent, two minutes, adding the clove of garlic for the last minute, so it does not burn.

Add the carrot and sauté for two minutes.

Add zucchini and sauté for two minutes.

Add the diced tomato. If you like the flavor, you can buy diced tomato with garlic, basil and oregano in the market. If you buy plain diced tomato, at this point, add a pinch of dried oregano. Use a light touch, because oregano can overpower the dish.

Add a teaspoon of Gourmet Garden parsley paste and a teaspoon of Gourmet Garden basil paste for the last few minutes of cooking.

Add the chicken broth and the pasta and cook for twenty minutes.

Drain the beans and rinse them. Add the beans, stir and warm the beans for five minutes.

For the Purée

Allow the soup to cool.

Stir the soup thoroughly and add one cup of soup to the small pitcher of a blender.

Pulse five times to break down the noodles and the beans.

Purée until smooth. This makes a purée of a good consistency.

To bind one serving of the soup, use a half scoop or a half pump of instant thickener and combine well. Wait several minutes before serving for the thickener to reach its maximum thickening potential.

For batch cooking: If you are puréeing the whole pot of soup for freezing in individual portions, use the large pitcher of a blender. Fill only 2/3 full. Make sure the soup is cool.

Pulse a few times to break down beans and noodles. Purée until smooth.

Divide the soup into individual storage containers. Label each container with the date created and the USE BY date. Store in the freezer.

Mark on the white board.

Won Ton Soup at Home

Calories	237
Fat	5.5 g.
Saturated Fat	1.5 g.
Sodium	930 mg.
Sugar	4 g.
Carbohydrate	36 g.
Fiber	4 g.
Protein	21 g.

Prep Time: 10 minutes
Cook Time: 4 minutes
Level: Easy
Serves 4

This is fast and easy and purées beautifully. It is a light soup and is delicious chilled in summer. It contains protein, green veggie and carbs.

Ingredients

- 1 quart lower sodium chicken broth, homemade or store bought
- 1 package FG brand gluten free potstickers, chicken or vegetable
- 1 half bunch fresh spinach
- 8 oz. roast loin of pork (from recipe above)
- 1 inch slice ginger
- 2 scallions sliced thinly on the diagonal
- Several shots of lower sodium soy sauce to taste

Directions

Bring the chicken broth to a boil and turn it down to a simmer

Add the ginger and scallions

Add the spinach

Prepare potstickers according to instructions, 90 seconds microwave.

Slice the pork into matchsticks

For the Purée

Allow the soup to cool. Remove the slice of ginger with a spider

Allow the potstickers to cool. Place the pork into the bowl of a mini food processor.

Pulse five times to break up pork. Purée with 2 tablespoons of broth for 10 seconds..

Place four potstickers in the bowl of the mini food processor.

Pulse four times to break down.

Purée with the pork until smooth, about 10 seconds.

Place one cup of soup into the pitcher of a blender, including scallions and spinach Blend until completely smooth.

Add the puréed pork and potstickers and blend until fully combined, about 10 seconds.

Add one pump or one scoop of instant thickener and blend until thoroughly combined. If necessary, add additional thickener until the soup is the correct consistency for the level of the NDD diet.

Divide into four individual servings. This freezes well.

Chawan Mushi
(Japanese Egg Custard Soup)

Prep Time: 10 minutes
Cook Time: 12 minutes
Level: Medium
Serves 1

PER SERVING

Calories	86
Fat	5 g.
Saturated Fat	1 g.
Sodium	238 mg.
Sugar	0 g.
Carbohydrate	1 g.
Fiber	0 g.
Protein	10 g.

This is an adaptation of a Japanese egg custard soup. It is steamed, so you will need a couple of small cups, Japanese tea cups. Chawan means teacup in Japanese. You could also use ramekins for making individual soufflés. Available in most supermarkets or kitchen stores. I use the Creuset brand.

The custard is very soft and delicate, so I am advising puréeing the ingredients before you steam the custard. This way, the pieces of chicken, shrimp and mushroom are already of purée consistency and the egg custard is very soft. Traditionally the soup has all the ingredients added whole to the custard. The proteins are already cooked. The puréed scallion and mushroom will have enough time to cook in the steaming.

Equipment: Steaming is an excellent cooking technique for the dysphagia kitchen. This cooking method gives moist tender protein and softens vegetables while preserving their nutritional content.

I have three go to appliances for easy steaming of vegetables and protein as well as puddings, custards and cakes in the dysphagia kitchen. There is also a fourth that can be adapted for steaming.

These appliances are well worth the initial investment. They are versatile in terms of the amounts that can be prepared in them. They pay for themselves because you don't have to buy commercially prepared food and takeout food, Standard kitchen equipment for steaming of custard would be a steaming rack in the bottom of a stock pot over two inches of water at the simmer. Pot should have a lid. Water should simmer, not boil.

I love the Wolfgang Puck 3-tiered steamer. You may use only one layer of this appliance for steaming small portions.

You may also use two or three layers. This means you can steam a protein, a carb and a vegetables in a parchment paper packet or an aluminum foil packet at the same time.

I have a Ninja multi-cooker that has a steaming rack and a steam setting. This will allow for the steaming of one or more portions.

I just acquired a Ming Tsai Turboconvection oven that has a steaming rack and a steaming function. This would also steam one or more portions. Early testing has yielded good results.

All three of these appliances have time set functions and easy programming. The ability to set a timer frees up kitchen time and energy. All three are easy cleanup.

The mini rice cooker will also steam one serving. If you use this appliance for steaming the custard soup, please place a small steaming rack in the bottom of the rice cooker, add an inch of water and turn on the rice cooker. You will have to time it for twelve minutes as the chip in the device may not read because of the rack. With a twelve minute cook time, you may have to add additional water because this device does not have a clock setting.

For the time-challenged caregiver or cook in a home healthcare setting, one may steam from frozen.

This is a very soothing dish.

Ingredients
- 1 cup broth (chicken, vegetable or even dashi (Japanese broth) from the whole foods store or Asian market)
- 1 tsp. lower sodium soy sauce
- 2 eggs
- 4 tablespoons of mushrooms
- 4 oz. cooked chicken breast meat cut into cubes (leftover chicken is ideal)
- 4 shrimp cooked
- 2 scallions very thinly sliced
- 2 tablespoons julienned carrot sticks

Directions
Purée the chicken, shrimp, scallions and carrots, using a little of the broth if need be. Whisk the eggs until combined. Add the broth, the soy sauce and the puréed vegetables.

Pour the mixture into a ramekin. Add about two inches of water to the bottom of a stock pot with a steaming rack set in it. I use an automatic slow cooker that has a steaming rack in it, one which will allow the lid to close. Water should simmer, not boil. Cover pot with a lid. Steam for 12 minutes, until eggs are set. Toothpick will come out clean when custard is done.

Allow to cool, as patients with swallowing difficulties should eat food that is only warm, not hot. Close to room temperature, but with enough warmth to give a feeling of satisfaction.

For the Purée

If the veggies and proteins are thoroughly puréed before adding to the custard, there is no need to purée this dish.

Custard is of pudding consistency. Make sure this is cleared by your healthcare provider for your level of the National Dysphagia Diet.

Mushroom Barley Soup

Prep Time: 10 minutes
Cook Time: 1 hour
Level: Easy
Serves 4

PER SERVING

Calories	261
Fat	6 g.
Saturated Fat	1 g.
Sodium	181 mg.
Sugar	3 g.
Carbohydrate	46 g.
Fiber	9 g.
Protein	9 g.

I make my mushroom barley soup with chicken or vegetable stock, rather than beef stock. Use beef stock if you prefer the flavor.

Ingredients

- 1 pound quartered mushrooms of your favorite variety. I use Baby Bellas for flavor.
- 4 scallions, sliced or half an onion, yellow or white, sliced
- 2 carrots, sliced into half moons
- 1 cup pearl barley, rinsed
- 1 quart chicken stock, lower sodium, homemade or store bought
- 1 tbsp. olive oil

Directions

Sauté scallions in olive oil 1 minute.

Add carrots, sauté one minute.

Add mushrooms and cook until they get some color and get soft. If mushrooms absorb all the liquid, add water or stock a tablespoon at a time so pan does not dry out. I add a shot of lower sodium soy sauce as it pairs beautifully with mushrooms and also with chicken stock.

Add barley and swirl in the bottom of your soup pot to get the grain coated with oil.

Add stock. Cook for thirty minutes at a simmer until barley is soft. When that happens, soup is done.

About five minutes into the cooking, you will notice a light foam forming on the surface of the soup. This is normal. It consists of impurities within the veggies. Skin the foam off using a tablespoon and discard.

For the Purée

This soup purées beautifully and also freezes beautifully. Served with a salad, this makes a light lunch.

When the soup is cooled, place a cup of soup in the bowl of a mini food processor or the small pitcher of a blender.

Purée until smooth.

If necessary, add a scoop or a pump of instant thickener to achieve the correct consistency for the prescribed level of the NDD

Tomato Cucumber Salad with Red Onion

Prep Time: 15 minutes
Level: Easy
Serves 2

PER SERVING

Calories	143
Fat	14 g.
Saturated Fat	2 g.
Sodium	26 mg.
Sugar	2 g.
Carbohydrate	5 g.
Fiber	1 g.
Protein	1 g.

Ingredients

- 1 medium tomato, quartered, seeded
- ½ hothouse cucumber, peeled, seeds removed, sliced
- ¼ small red onion, diced
- 3 tbsp. vinaigrette dressing, homemade or store bought

For the Purée

Equipment: For vegetable salads, I use the nutrient extractor, the NutriBullet or the NutriNinja.

Cut tomato in half and clean out seeds. Chop and add to the small cup of the nutrition extractor.

Add the rest of the ingredients. Extract for 10 seconds then test the texture. Extract an extra 10 seconds, if necessary. The vegetables will be liquefied. If there are any fibers, run the liquid through a mesh sieve with a silicone spatula.

Add a tablespoon of instant thickener and test the thickness for your level of the NDD. If needed, add more thickener a teaspoon at a time. Combine well. Allow to set up in the refrigerator for 10 minutes.

Vinaigrette Dressing

A standard vinaigrette is one part vinegar to three parts oil, but since my mother likes less oil, I use a 2-to-1 ration of oil to vinegar. Salt and white pepper to taste. Mixes the salad dressing with a fork until it is well combined.

Diane's Hummus

Yield: Two cups, 4 half-cup servings

PER SERVING

Calories	207
Fat	9 g.
Saturated Fat	1 g.
Sodium	287 mg.
Sugar	1 g.
Carbohydrate	27 g.
Fiber	6 g.
Protein	7 g.

Hummus, the Middle Eastern purée of chick peas, has made its way into the American supermarket. You can find it in the deli section of many groceries.

This is an excellent source of protein. It can be used as a substitute for mayonnaise in a number of salads. The homemade version is easy to make. The good part is that you can adjust the flavor to taste, adding more lemon or garlic, as you like it. Check store bought hummus for salt content, as it may sometimes be high, for those who are watching sodium.

This is quick and easy. I like to use it as the base for a chopped Greek salad with red onion, tomato, cucumber and olives. You can add a little vinaigrette dressing, also homemade. For chopped Greek salad, use a nutrition extractor such as a Ninja or NutriBullet. Add 3/4 cup of salad to the extractor and buzz for 10 seconds. Check to see if salad is liquefied. Add ½ cup store bought hummus and buzz for five to 10 seconds.

Ingredients

- 1 can garbanzo beans (15 oz.) drained, rinsed, liquid reserved. Also called chick peas
- ¼ cup tahini or sesame paste (available in supermarkets or in whole foods stores)
- Juice of two lemons
- 2 cloves of garlic (or to taste)
- ¼ tsp. salt, 1/8 tsp. white pepper
- 2 tablespoons reserved liquid from beans or water

For the Purée

Place all the ingredients in bowl of Ninja and pulse five times to get it going. Purée until smooth, about 10 seconds." Taste for seasoning. Adjust to taste.

Store in airtight container with label stating date. Keeps for four weeks in fridge.

Tuna Avocado Salad

Prep Time: 10 minutes
Level: Easy
Serves 2

Ingredients

- 1 can tuna, drained
- 1 avocado, sliced
- 2 tablespoons vinaigrette
- 1 tablespoon ranch dressing
- Salt and white pepper to taste
- 1 tablespoon fresh lemon juice

For the Purée

Place all ingredients in the bowl of a mini food processor. Pulse five times to incorporate.

Purée together. This is a smooth creamy salad with plenty of protein and good oils from the avocado. It makes a tasty tuna salad and can be served with a bowl of soup for a light dinner or for lunch. Nutrients for this recipe were calculated using the lower sodium tuna.

Variation

If you like, you can substitute crab meat for the tuna, making the classic crab and avocado salad. I add a touch of lemon juice and a shot of hot sauce for crab. The lemon juice wakes it up.

You can also add a tablespoon of hummus to this recipe to boost the nutrition.

For the Bread Component

In the bowl of a mini food processor, place four pieces of a cocktail loaf of seedless rye or pumpernickel bread. Add 2 tablespoons warm water and soak for several minutes until bread softens. You may use Italian bread or any good bread with the crusts removed.

Add ½ scoop or pump of instant thickener. Pulse to combine.

Place in a glass storage bowl and cover. Place in fridge or freezer for 10 minutes and allow to set up.

The bite is a half teaspoon of tuna avocado salad and a half teaspoon of puréed bread. Calories from bread not figured into the nutritional. See nutrition information on bread packaging.

Chunk Chicken Salad

PER SERVING

Calories	180
Fat	15 g.
Saturated Fat	2 g.
Sodium	70 mg.
Sugar	0 g.
Carbohydrate	1 g.
Fiber	1 g.
Protein	12 g.

Prep Time: 15 minutes
Level: Easy
Serves 2

Years ago, I had this chicken salad on Fire Island, bought from a specialty deli. It is very creamy and I always loved it.

Ingredients

- 1 cup leftover cooked chicken, cubed, about a pound (or poach one pound of chicken skinless and boneless chicken breast in lower sodium chicken broth for fifteen minutes at a simmer and allow to cool. Dice into one-inch cubes)
- 1 stalk celery, peeled with a vegetable peeler and diced into a small dice
- 2 tbsp. walnuts, chopped
- 2 tbsp. mayonnaise
- 2 tbsp. low fat sour cream
- 2 tbsp. Gourmet Garden parsley paste, or 2 tbsp. fresh parsley, minced
- Salt and white pepper to taste
- 2 tbsp. water for the purée

For the Purée

In the bowl of a mini food processor, place the chicken, the mayo, the water and the sour cream, Pulse five times until chicken is broken down. Add the remaining ingredients.

Purée together until smooth. Add water if needed for smooth consistency. If you poached your chicken, you can use 2 tbsp. of poaching liquid. Add a tablespoon of instant thickener to stabilize the purée and keep the liquid from separating.

Tip: Because I was cooking for a patient who had difficulty in swallowing, I always peeled the celery to get the strings off before the purée. It's an extra step, but it makes a better purée. Once can add all these ingredients to the small cup of a nutrient extractor such as the Ninja or the NutriBullet and extract until smooth. Stop after 10 seconds and check for the texture. Add another 10 seconds if needed

Red Beet Salad with Ranch Dressing

PER SERVING

Calories	90
Fat	6 g.
Saturated Fat	1 g.
Sodium	257 mg.
Sugar	6.5 g.
Carbohydrate	10 g.
Fiber	1 g.
Protein	1 g.

Prep Time: 10 minutes
Level: Easy
Serves 2

This was one of my mother's favorites. Some things are quickie and this is one of them.

I use a brand of picked beets that has a very low quantity of sugar. You want sweetness in this salad, to balance the sour taste of the vinegar on the palate. The ranch dressing tames the acid in the pickling juice, for the ease of the swallow. Check with your healthcare provider to make sure.

Equipment: The nutrition extractor is excellent for puréeing vegetables.

Ingredients

- 1 bottle sliced pickled beets, your favorite variety (I use Aunt Nellie's, six slices per serving)
- 2 tbsp. pickling liquid from jar, or 2 tbsp. water
- Optional: a half cup of very thinly sliced red onion to the pickled beets
- 6 tbsp. ranch dressing, your favorite kind (I use Ken's Steak House Buttermilk Ranch) when I do not have time to make it from scratch
- Salt and white pepper to taste

For the Purée

In the bowl of a mini food process, add the beets and 2 tbsp. of liquid, either pickling liquid or water.

Pulse four times to break down beets. Add the ranch dressing. Purée.

When smooth, add a pump or a scoop of instant thickener. Combine thoroughly.

This has wonderful flavor and color. It's pink. Remember, we eat with our eyes. A sure way out of patient boredom.

Sauces

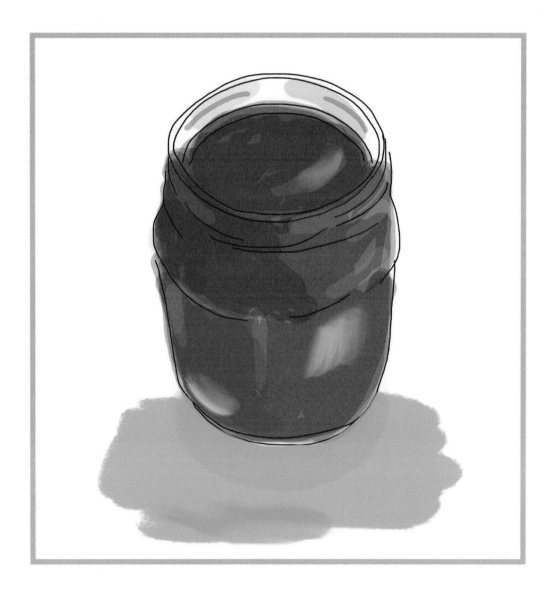

Pasta Sauce

Prep Time: 30 minutes
Cook Time: 3 hours
Level: Easy

In the world of Italian cooks, everyone has a favorite sauce. This is a variation on a family recipe that has been adapted. This is a meat sauce, but it can be made without meat. The object is to make enough to store in the freezer.

If the cook boils a pound of pasta, you can create individual servings for purée that consists of about ¾ a cup of cooked pasta for a regular appetite and either two meatballs, or a pork chop, or a sausage, depending on how you flavor your sauce. The pasta is stored in plastic freezer bags and can be defrosted in boiling water for a couple of minutes and then warmed in the individual serving of sauce with meatballs or meat, and then puréed. This makes a quickie dinner and is far more delicious than anything you can buy frozen and far healthier. The sauce freezes particularly well.

This is not difficult cooking. It involves the simplest and the best of ingredients, and the simplest of technique. I make a pot of sauce once every month or so, and it lasts. A good sauce is always a favorite with everyone.

This is not even a recipe. The sauce was absorbed by me, standing at my mother's side while she cooked. Everyone swooned and praised her meatballs and her sauce, and she had secrets that she imparted to me, as did my Aunt Lolly, my godmother, who was married to an Italian-American man, my uncle Chick. I know that some Italian Americans call the sauce "gravy" but in Aunt Lolly and Uncle Chick's house, it was always "sauce."

Start with the veggies. Sauté a diced onion and a couple of cloves of garlic.

If you want a Bolognese meat sauce, add carrot and celery, and sauté all together for 10 minutes. This is where you add the ground beef, pork or veal, or a combination of all three. You can add a quarter cup of red wine. You sauté all of this for about 10 minutes.

My mother always added a can of tomato paste at this point, thinned out with a little water. This adds thickness to the sauce, and gives it a depth of flavor. She would add a can of San Marzano tomatoes, crushed. A can of tomato purée. Two cans of tomato sauce. Simmer for two or three hours until the depth of flavor develops in the tomato.

Hint for the Sauce

You can sear a couple of pork chops and cook them two or three hours in the sauce until they fall off the bone. They flavor the sauce. The same is true for Italian sausage. My mother always added some sweet and some hot. The soft cooked pork chops are tender and can be puréed into the sauce. For sausage, buy the kind without the casing and add to the sauce. This also purées well.

Tip: You can start a sauce from scratch, using fresh tomatoes, garlic and onions, and fresh herbs, but that cooks only for a few minutes and is typically made in small batches.

Tip: An alternative to making your own is to buy good store bought sauce. I buy those whose first ingredient is plum tomatoes or any other tomato, rather than tomato purée. The flavor is better.

The Meatball

See Recipe for Diane's Turkey Meatballs

For the Purée

In a skillet, add one cup of sauce, one half cup pasta and two meatballs, then sprinkle with good parmesan cheese. Buy a wedge and grate it. Do not use the stuff off the shelf with the fillers. While warming the dish through, add the fresh parsley or the fresh basil or both. Add a few red pepper flakes if you like them.

A serving is one cup of sauce, three quarters cup of cooked pasta, two turkey meatballs.

This sauce freezes beautifully in two cup containers.

Diane's Pesto

Prep Time: 15 minutes
Level: Easy

PER SERVING

Calories	116
Fat	12 g.
Saturated Fat	2 g.
Sodium	83 mg.
Sugar	0 g.
Carbohydrate	1 g.
Fiber	1 g.
Protein	1 g.

This is very easy to make and will flavor a soup, a salad, as well as any number of pasta dishes, such as a pasta prima vera made with sautéed veggies.

Ingredients

- 2 cups fresh basil leaves, from your herb garden or from the supermarket, washed and patted dry in a paper towel, stems removed
- 2 large cloves garlic
- ¼ teaspoon sea salt
- ¼ cup Parmigiano reggiano
- ¼ cup pine nuts, raw for a creamy texture
- ½ cup extra virgin olive oil

For the Purée

In a food chopper or mini-food processor, place the garlic cloves and the sea salt, and give them a spin until the garlic becomes minced.

Add basil leaves and give a second spin until basil is finely chopped.

Add one half of the olive oil and give a spin.

Add the pine nuts and Parmigiano and the rest of the olive oil and spin until you have the consistency of a sauce. Give the pesto an extra buzz to purée the pine nuts rather than leave them crunchy as in traditional pesto.

If you like more olive oil, for use on pasta, add it. If the person with the swallowing difficulty prefers less garlic, by all means reduce the amount of garlic in the sauce. The basil is the thing. It is fragrant and loaded with flavor. If the person with the swallowing difficulty does not like raw garlic, you can sauté it for a minute until translucent and take away the raw taste or you can eliminate it and make a basil and olive oil herb sauce with Parmigiano or Romano cheese.

Store pesto in a container in refrigerator for several weeks. Freezes very well.

Makes about ¾ cup. Serving size for ½ cup cooked pasta is 2 tbsp.

Tip: For a quickie dinner on a night when you are strapped for time, prepare store bought cheese tortellini according to package directions, cooking the little cheese-filled tortoises until they are soft, and not al dente. Add a tablespoon of the pesto to a one cup serving of pasta. You have an instant entrée.

You can add cooked chicken or sautéed veggies to expand the dish. Serve with the tomato, olive and arugula salad and grilled veggies and you have a meal.

Tip: Add a teaspoon of pesto to the minestrone soup for added depth of flavor. Use in store bought tomato soup, in pasta sauce, on grilled fish when puréeing, in pasta with sautéed veggies and shrimp.

Note: For a quickie vinaigrette, use two parts olive oil, one part red wine vinegar, one teaspoon Dijon mustard for emulsifying, and salt and white pepper to taste. Stir with a fork or blend in blender. You can add finely minced shallots and a clove of finely minced garlic if this suits your palate.

Use any vinegar that suits your palate. I like Japanese rice vinegar for a very light dressing. There are many specialty vinegars such as sherry vinegar and champagne vinegar and each of them imparts a slightly different flavor. Lemon juice may be substituted for vinegar, the classic citronette. This happens to be my personal favorite, because I love lemon. It brightens up any dish.

Desserts

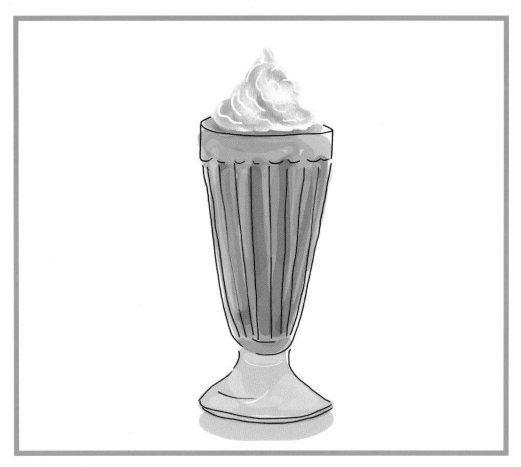

Recently I discovered from conversations with two eminent healthcare professionals that there was a real need for nutritionally dense desserts for the person with swallowing difficulties. In answer to this need, I offer the Deconstructed Dessert. These are quickie desserts that make use of high quality ingredients but are a shortcut. If you have a favorite ingredient, please feel free to substitute. Let these recipes be your inspiration and create using the basic proportions and methods. In other words, How to Make a Cake or Pie without Making a Cake or Pie. The bottom line is flavor.

Chocolate Cake with Frosting

PER SERVING

Calories	221
Fat	7 g.
Saturated Fat	1 g.
Sodium	82 mg.
Sugar	20 g.
Carbohydrate	38 g.
Fiber	1 g.
Protein	5 g.

Prep Time: 10 minutes
Cook Time: 10 minutes
Level: Intermediate
Yield: 6 jumbo cupcakes

Who does not like chocolate cake? It is probably American's favorite cake. (Those with food allergies, and please excuse.)

This recipe uses a high quality box cake mix. I use a cupcake maker appliance. I bake off the recipe. I store the extra cupcakes in the freezer. Below I give the shortcut recipe from a very high quality mix, for those who are time-challenged. This beats the taste of anything you can buy that is commercially prepared. The texture is tender. It is also cheaper, in addition to tasting better. It stores beautifully in either fridge or freezer. See my tips below.

Ingredients

- 2 cups whole wheat pastry flour
- 2 tsp. baking powder
- ½ tsp. salt
- 6 tbsp. cocoa
- 1 egg
- ⅓ cup oil
- ¾ cup honey
- 1 tsp. vanilla
- 1 cup milk
- 1 cup boiling water
- 1 tbsp. hot fudge sauce for lava filling

The boiling water makes the cocoa into a chocolate-y liquid.

Directions

Mix up the cake batter according to package directions.

Line the cupcake maker with a strip of parchment paper folded over. Add a cupcake liner. (The parchment allows you to lift the cupcake out easily.)

Using an ice cream scoop, fill the cupcake liners to 3/4 full.

Close the lid of the cupcake maker and plug it in and turn it on. I do not preheat for the first batch.

Allow the cupcake maker to go through its cycle, about 18 minutes.

After fifteen minutes, check on the cupcakes.

Test for doneness by inserting a toothpick into the center of the cupcake. When it comes out clean, the cupcake is done.

Lift out using the parchment paper sling. Place on a plate and allow to cool.

When the cupcake maker cools down, repeat the process. Add the parchment sling, add the cupcake liner, fill the cupcake liner 3/4 full with an ice cream scoop, close the lid and bake.

Allow cupcakes to cool.

Make a batch of the Most Delicious Chocolate Frosting.

Use 2 tablespoons of frosting for each cupcake.

If there is any leftover frosting, put it in a storage dish, label it and freeze it. To defrost, place in fridge for two hours. To use this frosting as a dipping sauce for puréed pound cake, add 1 tablespoon of warm water for 2 tablespoons of frosting and stir until it reaches pudding consistency. Add more warm water if necessary.

The short cut: I can make anything from scratch, but sometimes I don't have time. My shortcut is a fantastic chocolate organic cake mix from the European Gourmet Bakery Organics Line. I buy it at the whole foods store. The chocolate flavor is excellent. I make it according to package directions in a Wolfgang Puck cupcake maker. The mix yields six jumbo cupcakes. A serving size is one half of one cupcake plus two tablespoons of frosting.

For the Purée

Take one half of one jumbo cupcake and break it up in the bowl of a mini food processor.

Add 2 tablespoons of the Most Delicious Chocolate Frosting.

Add ½ cup of softened vanilla frozen yogurt or several tablespoons of milk

Pulse several times to break up the cake and then purée until smooth.

To bind the dessert, add instant thickener.

Equipment: I use the Wolfgang Puck cupcake maker because the cupcake is truly jumbo, with a deep well. This gives a moist product that is excellent for purée. One does not want fine crumbs in the purée as this is difficult for swallowing.

Tip: For a special zing in the purée, use a teaspoon of seedless, low sugar raspberry jam. This mimics the flavor of Black Forest Cake.

Tip: I use a cupcake maker appliance for this cake. For those who do not wish to use a cupcake maker: Bake off the cake in two 9 -inch cake pans, following package directions. Frost as you would a regular cake, with a layer of frosting in the middle and a layer of frosting on top. Freeze all the portions not used right away, using the wrapping techniques of plastic wrap, aluminum foil and placed in a freezer tight storage dish in single servings. A serving is a slice. Purée instructions are the same for one piece of cake as for one half a cupcake.

Tip: Taking a hint from the baker at my local supermarket, I wrap the cupcakes in plastic wrap, then in aluminum foil, and store them in a plastic freezer container with a tight silicon seal. Cupcakes remain fresh when defrosted and used within two weeks. Thaw for two hours in the fridge or one hour on the countertop. Fifteen second in the microwave. Frosting can be mixed up in five minutes and added to cupcakes after they thaw.

Most Delicious Chocolate Frosting

PER SERVING

Calories	33
Fat	2 g.
Saturated Fat	1 g.
Sodium	5 mg.
Sugar	2 g.
Carbohydrate	3 g.
Fiber	0 g.
Protein	0 g.

This is an easy frosting, simple to make, not too sweet. It has great texture because of the silkiness of the sour cream.

You could also use buttermilk, the great staple of the Southern kitchen. Use it to top the cupcakes before you wrap them up to freeze them. One tablespoon of frosting per cupcake. The cupcake will be puréed with the frosting using ½ cup of frozen yogurt softened.

Ingredients

- ¼ cup Nocciolata, organic hazelnut spread with cocoa and milk,
- ¼ cup to ¼ cup low fat sour cream

Directions

Add ingredients to bowl and blend with a spoon to frosting consistency.

Frost each cupcake.

For the Purée

Use one half of one jumbo cupcake plus two tablespoons of frosting.

Break up the cupcake in the bowl of a mini food processor.

Add one half cup of softened vanilla frozen yogurt or any flavor you like.

If you do not wish to use softened ice cream or frozen yogurt, use several tablespoons of milk to purée the cupcake and frosting.

Pulse a few times to break up.

Purée. Add more softened yogurt, if necessary.

Add instant thickener to stabilize the cake and ice cream.

Tip: The Ultimate Quickie Recipe: Buy a store bought chocolate cake and purée each slice according to directions. Freeze extra servings according to directions.

Tip: Nocciolata is available at whole foods stores in small jars and from Wal-Mart Online in larger containers. I use it because unlike a popular brand, Nocciolata has no trans-fats. The philosophy of Essential Purée is to use the finest ingredients and this one has superb flavor.

Apple Tart

Prep Time: 30 minutes
Cook Time: 40 minutes
Level: Easy

PER SERVING

Calories	108
Fat	4 g.
Saturated Fat	1 g.
Sodium	30 mg.
Sugar	15 g.
Carbohydrate	20 g.
Fiber	1 g.
Protein	1 g.

Ingredients

Filling

- 2 granny smith apples
- ¼ cup apple juice
- 2 tbsp. lemon juice
- ¼ cup honey
- ¼ tsp. cinnamon
- ⅛ tsp. salt
- ½ tsp. cornstarch or arrowroot

Crust

- 1 cup Ginger Snaps (Mi-Del brand has no trans fat)
- 1/3 cup warm water
- instant thickener

Directions

Filling: Peel and core apples and cut into even half moon slices. If the apples are all the same thickness, they will cook evenly.

Mix apple juice, lemon juice, honey, cinnamon and salt in a bowl. Add apples and mix thoroughly.

Add 1 tablespoon unsalted butter or non trans fat margarine to a saute pan. Add the mixture of apples and juice. Cook the filling over a low heat.

Add the cornstarch mixed with a tablespoon of cold water. Stir. Allow to come to the boil and cook for a minute as it thickens. This is your filling.

For the Purée

Crust: Break up one cup of ginger snaps in a bowl and add ¼ cup of warm water. Soak until soft. Add to the bowl of a mini food processor and purée for thirty seconds. Add one scoop or one pump of instant thickener and purée for 10 seconds.

This is your crust.

Divide the crust between two glass serving bowls, cover and place in the fridge for thirty minutes to set.

Filling: Add filling to bowl of mini food processor and purée until smooth. About 15 seconds.

Add 1 pump or 1 scoop instant thickener. Combine thoroughly.

Divide filling between two glass bowls.

Add layer of crust to each bowl of filling.

Cover and place in fridge.

For Serving

For warm apple pie, place in microwave and heat for 20 seconds at 50% power.

When serving, the spoon goes down through both layers. This is virtual apple pie.

Add a side dish of thickened vanilla ice cream for apple pie a la mode. The serving method is alternating bites or a combination bite, part thickened ice cream, part puréed pie.

For a holiday meal, I add a drizzle of St. Darfour's Organic Caramel Sauce. I heat two tablespoons in the microwave in a ceramic dish for 10 seconds to soften it. I drizzle it over the pie or over the ice cream. It has a sufficient thickness for the safe swallow. Just to be sure, check with your SLP or physician.

The apple pie freezes well in the covered glass dish. To serve from frozen, thaw in the fridge for two hours or on the counter top for one hour.

Strawberry Shortcake

Prep Time: 20 minutes
Fridge Time: 1 hour
Level: Easy

PER SERVING

Calories	240
Fat	20 g.
Saturated Fat	11 g.
Sodium	56 mg.
Sugar	10 g.
Carbohydrate	16 g.
Fiber	3 g.
Protein	2.5 g.

This is a quickie dessert, easy to assemble.

Equipment: Nutrient extractor such as a NutriBullet or NutriNinja..

Ingredients

- 1 piece store bought pound cake
- 1 cup fresh or frozen strawberries
- ¼ cup So CocoWhip whipped topping

For the Purée

For the shortcake: Break the piece of pound cake up and add to the bowl of a mini food processor. Add two tablespoons of warm milk or water and soak until soft. Pulse to break up, then purée until smooth. Add 1 tablespoon of instant thickener. Place the pound cake in a 4½ inch glass storage bowl and cover with lid. Place in fridge for one hour to set.

Prepare the strawberries: If using fresh strawberries, eliminate rough texture from fruit: clean off the tops and take out the white core. Clean off any bruised patches. Cut off the pointy tip. Frozen strawberries will already be cleaned.

Place fresh or frozen strawberries in the small cup of a NutriBullet or NutriNinja. Extract until liquefied. Strain the strawberries through a mesh sieve lined with cheesecloth, using a silicone spatula. Strawberry purée should be free of seeds. Add 1 tsp. of stevia or organic sugar or honey to taste. Combine thoroughly. This should yield 1/2 cup of strawberry purée. Thicken with instant thickener, enough for 4 oz. liquid until you reach the consistency for your level of the NDD.

Add this mixture to the bowl with the puréed cake.

Add 1 tablespoon of instant thickener to ¼ cup of whipped topping and combine thoroughly. Add this to the top of the strawberry shortcake in the glass bowl and cover. Place in fridge to chill.

Double the recipe to make two servings.

This freezes well. Defrost in fridge for two hours or on counter top for one hour.

Cathie G's Banana Cream Pie

Serves 4

PER SERVING

Calories	285
Fat	12 g.
Saturated Fat	6 g.
Sodium	145 mg
Sugar	20 g.
Carbohydrate	43 g.
Fiber	3 g.
Protein	3 g.

This was one of my mom's favorites, so I made a healthy version with no artificial flavorings and no preservatives or trans fats.

Ingredients

- 2 ripe bananas
- 1 tablespoon Smart Balance or Butter
- 1 teaspoon maple syrup
- 1 package banana or vanilla pudding made according to package directions. See below.
- 1 package shortbread, preferably good Scottish shortbread (Walker brand)
- ¼ cup So Coco Whip topping

Directions

This is a deconstructed pie intended for purée.

The pudding I use is European Gourmet Bakery Organics which I get at the natural food store. For non-dairy, can be made with full fat coconut milk.

Slice the bananas and melt the butter or shortening in a saucepan. Swirl the bananas in the butter and add the maple syrup. This should be warmed through and develops the rich flavor of the banana. Allow to cool.

For the Purée

Add 2 squares of shortbread to the bowl of a mini food processor. Add the butter and maple syrup mixture and soften cookies. Use 2 tablespoons warm milk if necessary. Pulse and then purée until smooth. Add 1 tablespoon instant thickener. Mix thoroughly. Add to glass storage bowl and set in fridge to set up. After one hour, add one half cup of pudding to the glass serving bowl.

Add 1 tablespoon of instant thickener to 4 tablespoons of the whipped topping, mix thoroughly and add to serving bowl. This is your pie.

Deelish.

One Last Note: Use the best kitchen tools. No matter the tool, here are your guidelines:

- Keep processing blades sharp and check routinely for blade condition. The rule of thumb is to replace the blade every six months if they are dulled by use.
- Do not fill a food processing bowl or a pitcher for a blender or extractor more than 2/3 full.
- Do not place hot foods in a plastic food processing bowl. Allow food to cool before processing.
- Foods process best when cold or cooled. Hot food can be cooled at room temperature to approximately 100°F.
- Cover and reheat hot foods in an oven or steamer after processing.
- To reheat food after purée, cover and place in a microwave at 50% power for 20 seconds, reheat in an oven-safe dish in a slow oven of 200 degrees for five minutes, reheat over low heat in a saucepan on a stovetop, or reheat for two minutes in the steamer rack of a multi-cooker or a steamer. Low and slow is the desired technique, no matter the cooking method.
- Glass containers are better for foods with instant thickeners. Gum thickeners stick to plastic.

What Kitchen Appliance should you use to purée? The blender is the most important tool for the dysphagia kitchen.

Please visit **EssentialPuree.com** for the latest reviews, recipes and tips.

The Science of Purée

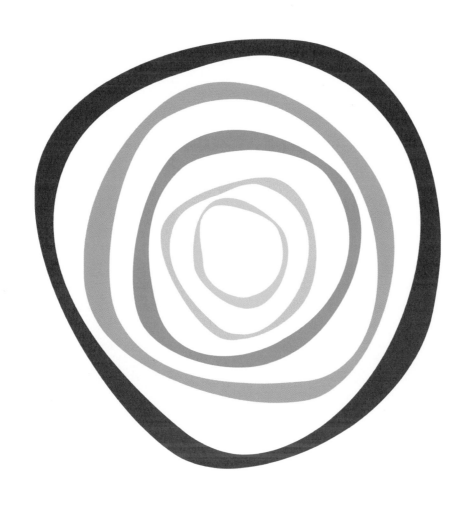

The National Dysphagia Diet

The National Dysphagia Diet (NDD) is the standard for dietary treatment of swallowing difficulties.

In 2002, the American Dietetic Association (now called the Academy of Nutrition and Dietetics) set the standards for the "National Dysphagia Diet: Standardization for Optimal Care."

As of the summer of 2015, the International Dysphagia Diet Standardization Initiative is working to standardize the terminology for food textures and liquid consistencies for use around the world, in all cultures and with all age groups.

The following terms apply to modification for foods and beverages. Your healthcare provider will determine which of these is appropriate for you.

There is no "one size fits all" diet. All diets must be created with the advice of one's healthcare providers, namely physicians and speech pathologists. Please consult your physician and speech therapist if you have any questions.

The National Dysphagia Diet Levels

If you've been told that you need to modify food textures, these are the standards:

- **The Regular Diet (Internationally known as "Level 7")**
  All foods are acceptable. Foods may be hard and crunchy, tough, crispy and may contain seeds, skins and husks. Persons on a regular diet have the ability to produce saliva and chew for as long as it takes for the food to form a cohesive "ball" (bolus) for safe swallowing. Mixed textures are no problem. Some patients have a temporary need for purée and return to the regular diet. Some patients remain on purée for reasons indicated in their own medical history.

- **Dysphagia Advanced Soft Diet (Internationally known as "Soft" or "Level 6")**
  Foods of "nearly regular" textures with the exception of very hard, sticky or crunchy foods. This texture requires chewing and tongue control. Foods should be tender and easy to break into pieces with a fork.

- **Dysphagia Mechanical Soft (Internationally known as "Minced and Moist" or "Level 5")**
Foods with a moist, soft texture. Ability to tolerate mixed textures needs to be assessed. Meats need to be chopped or ground. Vegetables need to be well cooked and easily chewed. Foods should be in small pieces (¼" or 5mm). No hard, chewy, fibrous, crisp or crumbly bits. No husk, seed, skins, gristle or crusts. No "floppy" textures such as lettuce and raw spinach. No foods where the juice separates from the solid upon chewing, like watermelon.
- **Dysphagia Puréed (Internationally known as "Extremely Thick" or "Level 4")**
All food should be puréed to a homogenous, cohesive, smooth texture. Foods should be "pudding-like" and hold its shape on a spoon. Contains no lumps. Not sticky. Puréed foods can be piped or molded and will not spread out if spilled. The prongs of a fork make a clear pattern when drawn across the surface of the purée.

Liquids

The Essential Purée Guidebook does not deal with the Liquid Diet, only liquids thickened as beverages, MEANING A NECTAR OR HONEY CONSISTENCY.

Your healthcare provider will determine if you may use any of the recipes in this book.

Here are the definitions of the three different consistency levels for the Liquid Diet:

- **Nectar Thick** liquids coat and drip off a spoon like a lightly-set gelatin. This consistency requires little more effort to drink than thin liquid. It is easier to control though the swallow than thin liquid and can flow through a straw or nipple. (Internationally known as "Slightly Thick" or "Level 1"
- **Honey Thick** liquids are thicker than "nectar thick" and flow off a spoon in a ribbon, like actual honey. This consistency allows for a more controlled swallow. This consistency is difficult to drink through a standard straw. (Internationally known as "Mildly Thick" or "Level 2")
- **Pudding Thick** liquids stay on a spoon in a soft mass but will not hold its shape. It pours slowly off a spoon and is sip-able. This consistency is difficult to draw though a wide-bore straw. (Internationally known as "Moderately Thick and Liquidized" or "Level 3")

For Clinicians: A Note from the Authors of the National Dysphagia Diet

The NDD authors stress that the categorization process is a work in progress and far from a perfect science, especially as applied to the individualized needs of each dysphagia patient.

While establishing liquid and food-related categorical protocols may help to create a standardized "starting point" to evaluate the specific needs of each patient, both the NDD task force and ASHA experts acknowledge that there is much research to be conducted and it should never be applied as a "one-size-fits-all" approach.

The International Dysphagia Diet Standardization Initiative (IDDSI) work group has taken up the challenge to look at the dysphagia diet from a global perspective.

They are a group of people from diverse professions including nutrition & dietetics, medicine, speech pathology, occupational therapy, nursing, patient safety, engineering, food science & technology from around the world who have come together to establish an international standardized terminology and definitions for texture modified foods and thickened liquids for persons with dysphagia.

In the next several years, clinicians just might see the next evolution of a the NDD.

The above information on the National Dysphagia Diet is the contribution of Laura Michael, a board member of the National Foundation of Swallowing Disorders and an ambassador to the ISSDI, the committee working on establishing international standards for the National Dysphagia Diet. Laura is the author of a clinical manual for caregivers that may be obtained from her website, DysphagiaSolutions.com

Thickeners

Instant Food Thickeners

Instant food thickeners are used to thicken liquids to the proper consistency for safe swallowing. They also bind purées so the components of a dish do not separate - they stabilize.

Instant food thickeners have come a long way in the last five years. Starch-based thickeners, like ThickIt, used to be the industry standard. Starch thickeners often add a starchy or pasty flavor to liquids. They make liquids cloudy and can only be used in certain liquids. Starch thickeners add carbohydrates and continue to thicken on standing, so they can be difficult to use and don't taste great.

Times have changed. New products have come on the market. Gum-based thickeners like Simply Thick and ThickenUp Clear, are now widely available.

Liquids thickened with these new gum-based thickeners are clear and taste just like the base beverage.

These thickeners do not add or alter flavor, mix easily into liquids, and can be used in all types of beverages (including alcohol and fizzy drinks). They do not continue to thicken upon standing.

These thickeners come in two forms: gel and powder. Powdered gum-based thickeners are no more expensive than starch thickeners. The containers are smaller because powdered gum-based thickeners are more concentrated than powdered starch thickeners.

Gel thickeners, like Simply Thick can be a bit more expensive than starch thickeners, but the higher cost may be worth it if you consume (and enjoy) the liquids you need for good health.

Simply Thick is a gel formula, gum-based thickener. It can be found at some pharmacies or online at simplythick.com.

ThickenUp Clear, Thick & Easy Clear, and SloDrinks are powdered gum-based thickeners.

ThickenUp Clear, a product of NestleNutrition, can be purchased at many Walgreen's stores or online. For more information: thickenupclear.com.

Thick & Easy Clear, from Hormel Health Labs, can be purchase online: homecarenutrition.com

SloDrinks produce beverage-specific gum-based thickeners in individual portions. You can purchase SloDrinks at Amazon.com.

How to Thicken Drinks

Hydration is important for the dysphagia patient, so it is important to have the ability to thicken many types of beverages.

There is an art to thickening liquids, including fruit juices, milk, coffee and tea, sodas and other carbonated beverages and alcoholic beverages. Don't be shocked. Not every dysphagia patient is alcohol-restricted.

One company has thought this need for hydration through and has created an excellent line of products for every type of beverage. It is called SlōDrinks.

This company was recommended to me by Laura Michael, the dysphagia care expert. They have a special line for beer, wine and bar drinks. If you are cleared for the consumption of alcoholic beverages, the product is sold on Amazon and also on their website.

I interviewed the founder of the company, Matthew Done. He explained the reason why there are different products for different drinks. Food science, dear readers, is important and it takes time.

"A drink's fat, sugar, temperature and pH levels affect a thickener's ability to thicken. . .As a result my company has different thickeners for different drinks. I think we are the only manufacturer to think this way, which is why it took 10 years to perfect our products!"

As Matthew explained, "It is essential to first make sure the thickener works in a drink and then calculate the amount required to make it a specific consistency."

Different thickeners for different liquids. That is why the full product line took 10 years to develope. SlōDrink thickeners are available in nectar and honey consistencies. The company also provides instructions for pudding consistency. You use less liquid rather than more thickener to get to the correct consistency for each individual.

The SlōDrinks website is informative. If you click on their YouTube link, you will find a How To video, with Matthew himself demonstrating how to use his company's products.

ALL LIQUIDS must be thickened for the dysphagia patient. This includes oral rinses and liquid medicines, such as cough medicines. It is easy to overlook liquids such as mouthwash and liquid medicines, but it is absolutely necessary.

SlōDrinks also makes a line of thickeners custom-tailored for taking medication, such as flu medication in hot or cold liquid. They have a second formula for pain medication and vitamins.

Pre-thickened Water and More

Producers are now making pre-thickened "clear" waters in both Nectar and Honey consistencies. These beverages have no flavor, are clear and reliably consistent.

Two brands to consider are:

Thick & Easy Clear water, from Hormel Health Labs, has a slight lemon flavor. It is available in Nectar and Honey consistency. You can purchase it as single-serve 4 oz. portions and 48 oz. bottles.

Thick & Easy also makes pre-thickened juices, coffee, iced tea and milk. Thick & Easy® products can be purchased online at homecarenutrition.com

ThickIt AquaCare H2O water, from Kent-Precision Foods, has no added flavors. It is available as Nectar and Honey consistency. It is available in 8 oz. bottles and 48 oz. bottles.

ThickIt AquaCare H2O makes a complete line of thickened juices, coffee and iced tea. Find ThickIt AquaCare H2O water in your grocery store or pharmacy. It is also available online: thickit.com/products/beverages

Reading Material

The Official Patient's Sourcebook on Dysphagia, published by Icon Health Publications, is available from icongroupbooks.com and various booksellers such as Amazon and Barnes & Noble.

American Heart Association's Nutrition Center
Heart.org/HEARTORG/GettingHealthy/NutritionCenter/Nutrition-Center_UCM_001188_SubHomePage.jsp

National Dysphagia Diet: What to Swallow
http://leader.pubs.asha.org/article.aspx?articleid=2292328

American Diabetes Association Diet Pages
Diabetes.org/food-and-fitness/food/what-can-i-eat/

Choose My Plate Nutrition Guide published by U. S. Department of Agriculture
ChooseMyPlate.gov
Click on videos for My Plate, Grains, Fruits and Veggies

Food Pyramid for Latin and Asian Cuisines published by The Mayo Clinic
MayoClinic.com/health/healthy-diet/NU00190

On Food Safety
Foodsafety.gov/keep/index.html

EssentialPuree.com

Be sure to visit our website where you can find:

- New Recipes
- Product Reviews
- Diane's latest blog posts: tips, tricks, tools and techniques
- ...and more!

To Order Copies of this Book

We offer discounts on bulk orders and for students. Please send an e-mail to orders@EssentialPuree.com for more information.

Acknowledgments

I would like to extend my sincere gratitude to the following people:

Dietitian Amy Tribolini, MS, RD, LD, for her work on the nutritional breakdowns of the recipes. Kathleen Oliver, the head Dietitian at Bayfront Medical Center, who helped me get the best products for my mom. Liza Zullig, Head Dietitian at God's Love We Deliver, for her support and for the amazing kitchen tour. Dr. Dee, nutritionist, chef and teacher, for her excellent suggestions and encouragement.

David Fagan, head Speech Language Pathologist at Fawcett Memorial Hospital, for his encouragement and support. Mary Spremulli, Speech Language Pathologist at Voice Aerobics, for her encouragement and suggestions.

Dr. Manuel Martinez, my mom's primary care physician, for his advice and support on all things affecting my mom's health care plan, including her diet and exercise, for many years. Dr. Amy Mellor, Neurologist, for her encouragement and appreciation.

Heidi Pines and Sue Block for their expertise in the fields of healthcare and startups in the food industry, respectively.

All the aides who cared for the late great Cathie G. Richard Wimmer for his advice, to Dana Wimmer for her friendship, and to Mike Lowe for his guidance. Csongor Daniel for his many years of excellent physical therapy for my mother. Rudy Pittaluga, my dad's protégé, for his unfailing support. Lewis Hall for his advice and support.

Jonathan Waller, the eminent Speech Language Pathologist and creator of DysphagiaCafe.com, for his enthusiastic support and encouragement.

Florida State Senator Nancy Detert, who thanked me for educating her on the importance of the issue of nutrition for the elderly and who promised to make her fellow legislators on the Committee for Children, Family and Elder Affairs aware of this issue.

18725175R00134

Printed in Great Britain
by Amazon